STEP UP YOUR GAME

The Revolutionary Program Elite Athletes Use to Increase Performance and Achieve Total Health

NARESH C. RAO, DO, FAOASM

SPORTS
PUBLISHING

Copyright © 2016 by Naresh C. Rao

All rights reserved. No part of this book may be reproduced in any manner without the express written consent of the publisher, except in the case of brief excerpts in critical reviews or articles. All inquiries should be addressed to Sports Publishing, 307 West 36th Street, 11th Floor, New York, NY 10018.

Sports Publishing books may be purchased in bulk at special discounts for sales promotion, corporate gifts, fund-raising, or educational purposes. Special editions can also be created to specifications. For details, contact the Special Sales Department, Sports Publishing, 307 West 36th Street, 11th Floor, New York, NY 10018 or sportspubbooks@skyhorsepublishing.com.

Sports Publishing® is a registered trademark of Skyhorse Publishing, Inc.®, a Delaware corporation.

Visit our website at www.sportspubbooks.com.

10 9 8 7 6 5 4 3 2 1

Library of Congress Cataloging-in-Publication Data is available on file.

Cover design by Tom Lau
Cover photo credit: Thinkstock by Getty Images/pretrelos

Interior photographs provided by Matt Simpkins

ISBN: 978-1-61321-830-3
Ebook ISBN: 978-1-61321-863-1

Printed in the United States of America

In memory of Neena and Sammy,
who are always there playing with me

CONTENTS

INTRODUCTION

Perfection is not attainable, but if we chase perfection we can catch excellence.

—Vince Lombardi

E lite athletes achieve their status because they can consistently perform at the highest levels of their chosen sport. They have dedicated their lives to the pursuit of perfection, and are justly rewarded. But like any celebrity, deep down we know that they are just human, and basically, no different than us. Or are they?

Over the past fifteen years I have come to know and treat hundreds of elite athletes ranging from professionals to Olympic superstars, triathletes and marathoners, as well as a full range of weekend warriors, and I've learned exactly what separates superstars from the rest of us, despite our best efforts. First, elite athletes benefit from both nature and nurture. Many have some type of genetic predisposition that is ideal for their chosen sport. This may have been recognized at an early age: long limbs ideal for swimming, a naturally strong core for wrestling, a limberness for diving or gymnastics. Elite athletes also have an innate, fierce determination and can go after their goals single-mindedly. Some put in the requisite 10,000 hours toward mastery when they were kids, such as Tiger Woods or Maria Sharapova, while others came to their sport later in their development, like Michael Jordan, who spent much of his youth pursuing baseball.

At the same time, these top athletes clearly respond to nurture: the positive feedback they get from achieving the gold medal or the trophy or the fame pushes them to work harder, put in more hours, and perfect their skills. What's more, they all seem to love what they do; they live and breathe their sport. It's an exciting, integral part of their everyday lifestyle.

While the media often picks up on the backstories that reveal the talent or relentless effort that propelled these athletes to greatness, this illusion of singularity often leaves us believing that sports icons accomplish their goals alone. But nothing could be further from the truth. In fact, the real secret behind every uber-successful athlete is their entourage.

Today's elite athletes know that while skill and consistent practice are ingredients to their success, the only way they can reach their goals is through the creation of an individualized, comprehensive program that takes into account every aspect of wellness optimization, ranging from monitoring health to improving nutrition, a goal-based training regimen, and a protocol for recovering from and preventing injury. They also recognize that their mental game is just as important as their physical one, and they proactively address their motivational, psychological, and spiritual needs. In short, the athletes who are at the top of their game know that if they want to improve in some way—whether it's their accuracy at the goal, time at the finish line, or dependability of play—they need to take all of these aspects into consideration every single day.

The only way they can accomplish this enormous task while concentrating all of their efforts on improving their performance is by delegating these facets of training to experts. For the very lucky few who have unlimited funds from either corporate sponsors, university backers, or a dedicated family, their wellness program is carefully orchestrated by nine distinct professionals who, more often than not, include:

- Team Physician
- Physical Therapist
- Trainer
- Dietitian
- Coach

- Competitor
- Role/Model Hero
- Psychologist
- Spiritual Leader

These roles form the core idea behind this program. And I'm not alone in thinking this way. In a 2015 *New York Times* article, Yael Averbuch, a midfielder for F. C. Kansas City (of the National Women's Soccer League) and the US Women's National Team, wrote, "Over the years, I have devised methods of training and improving on my own. But I have learned that there are aspects of getting to the next level that I cannot tap into independently. For this, it is best to find an expert."

The goal of *Step Up Your Game* is to provide the best practices of each of these nine roles, based on the latest research. The truth is, you can take on many of these roles yourself, and in this book you will learn exactly how to do so. In effect, you will be able to organize your training in a completely systematic way just like an elite athlete would, regardless of your level of expertise.

By integrating this program into your existing fitness routine, you will take full ownership of your training, and even more importantly, you will remove some of the stress that often hampers outcomes. For instance, my network approach to wellness will alleviate feelings of frustration and loneliness when you are facing a particular challenge, because you will have expert advice to answer your issues right at your fingertips. By taking a proactive approach to your training, you'll have the best chance for achieving your goals with greater focus and fewer excuses. Best of all, by following this program you will be able to step up your game because both your body and mind will be in the best position to attain success. You'll finally break through the plateaus, set higher goals, and get to the next level while minimizing your risk of injury, burnout, or overtraining.

This unique approach has been enormously beneficial for the San Diego State University athletics department, Oracle/BMW Racing's

America's Cup Team, USA Water Polo (including the 2012 Gold Medal Women's Olympic team) and thousands of my private clients. The *Step Up Your Game* methodology works whether you participate in team sports or individual competition, and applies to all athletic pursuits: triathlete, gym rat, tennis player, swimmer, golfer, and more. The reason its reach is so broad and flexible is that it is organized by core lifestyle principles many athletes intuitively grasp. We know we are supposed to eat right, exercise, and take care of our bodies and minds. Yet without specific guidelines, I've found that few people actually put these practices into action, or concentrate on only a few to the detriment of the others. So while you may already be incorporating some of my suggestions into your training, unless you are doing all of the work in concert, you won't be able to achieve the results you desire.

I have also found that it is one of the best ways to not only train better, but to bring the fun back to your sport as well. When you know that all of the necessary systems have been put in place and that you are covering every aspect of training, you will finally be able to relax and enjoy the entire experience as you work to achieve your healthiest, most athletic self.

The Step Up Your Game Philosophy

Combining my passions for science and athletics were integral for developing this program and for framing my medical practice. I've always thought of myself as an athlete. I played competitive football, basketball, and tennis in high school, and club water polo in college. I completed my first marathon in 2006, and have continued to play tennis and water polo throughout the years. I also coach water polo and swimming at the New York Athletic Club's Saturday Morning Program, which introduces children to various sports in the Olympic tradition.

I can trace the roots of this program back to my youth. In the summer of 1986 I was fourteen years old and attended the Big Orange Basketball Camp at the Carrier Dome in Syracuse, New York. Derrick

Coleman, the future New Jersey Net and then high school phenom was on center court right near me showing off his amazing skills to the recruiters, while Syracuse University's legendary head coach Jim Boeheim was scouting the talent. A strength and conditioning coach had us run suicide drills to enhance our speed, endurance, and agility, and a physician was on hand in case anyone got injured. Even Charles Barkley, one of my basketball idols at that time and then All-Star NBA player, came to the camp and gave a talk to inspire us. I realized then that each of these professionals was there to help me improve. I expected that a coach and the boys in my age group would constitute my team, but to have access to all of these experts, along with my basketball heroes, was more than a luxury: it was exactly what I needed to take my performance from just average to the next level.

I turned out to be correct. I focused on their messages and worked harder that summer than I ever did before. Because of this discipline, every year I got a little bit better. I was able to effortlessly switch from one seasonal sport to another. In college, I started playing water polo. My close friends Craig Pizer and Matt Kaplan had started an intercollegiate water polo club at Colgate University. It was the hardest sport I had ever played, and it transformed my mind and my body. I was still applying the methods I learned at basketball camp, and by the end of the first season I was in the best shape of my life. What's more, I recognized that the discipline I adopted carried over to the classroom, the laboratory, and eventually to medical school.

My first decision was to forgo the traditional, allopathic (MD) medical training that my father had undergone, and instead study to be an osteopathic (DO) physician. I was attracted to the DO degree because of its unique approach in taking the whole person into account, including physical, emotional and spiritual components, instead of concentrating on specific symptoms or illnesses. Within this context I decided to focus on primary care, where I could continue to practice a preventive approach to avoiding disease, averting injury, and helping patients achieve their highest performance based on the latest research. My training in Family Medicine integrates the biological, clinical, and behavioral sciences to provide continuing and comprehensive health care for all ages, sexes, each organ system, and every disease. I've been trained to pay special attention to my patients' lives within the context of their family and the community. This combination of skills allows me to treat the whole person rather than treating a specific illness or set of symptoms, which is a very different approach than other specialties practice within medicine.

In order to marry my interests of sports and medicine, I completed a fellowship in sports medicine in 2002, with the hope of becoming a team physician. During this time I learned many aspects of sports medicine, ranging from how to direct medical care for various teams at San Diego State University to acting as the medical director for San Diego's Bayfair World Series of Powerboat Racing—those high speed boats that move well over 200 miles per hour.

One of my first experiences during my fellowship was to cover a clinic for Oracle BMW Racing's America's Cup campaign. I introduced myself to the athletic trainer, ready to take care of some of the top sailors in the world. But the first patient to walk in was one of the sailor's wives who was five months pregnant and was complaining of feeling light-headed. At that moment I remembered I had delivered fifty babies in my training, and I said to myself, *Thank God I am a family physician!*

As I went from game to game, sport to sport, boat to dock, I noticed for the first time that all of the elite athletes I treated had one thing in common. In order for them to perform at their highest level, they were never alone: they all required an entourage.

I remember standing on the sidelines of a Division I NCAA football game for San Diego State University, under the lights in Qualcomm Stadium. One of their star starting linebackers was having back issues just as he was supposed to take the field. The athletic trainers and sports doctors, both primary care and orthopedic, were attending to him but were unable to get rid of his pain. Even though I was just in training, I offered to see what I could do. I laid the player on the ground and then proceeded to perform a technique called osteopathic manipulative treatment. After five minutes of working on him, I had him get up and test out his back. Sure enough, my therapy had worked! The player ran onto the field, and on the very next play he got an interception, which completely changed the momentum of the game. The head team orthopedist later came up to me and said, "Naresh, that was your interception: great job."

That was the moment when I knew exactly what I was intended to do. The similarities between experiencing the support roles when I was a young athlete and witnessing them in action at the college and national team level were striking. For example, at the basketball camp the strength and conditioning coach taught us plyometrics in order for us to learn how to jump higher; the same role would be instrumental in teaching a San Diego State football player how to bench press 300 pounds. This is how I know that every athlete can improve their performance by taking charge of their training and inspecting every aspect of their program to see that key roles are present and working synergistically.

The year after that I completed the first ever Wellness Medicine Fellowship. This program applied everything I had been taught about sports medicine for the average patient, including myself. It turned out to be one of the biggest challenges I had ever faced because I had to live the message. I completed a specialized cardiovascular rehab rotation with Dorian Dugmore, PhD, at the Adidas Wellness Center in Manchester, England. Back home, I went to retreats, including personal growth workshops (very California), medical workshops, and even relationship workshops with my wife. I took spirituality workshops at Innerpath Retreats in Tucson, Arizona, and I learned about addiction at a Professional in Residence Program at the Betty Ford Center. Suddenly, I was no longer viewing myself through the lens of "doctor" or "post-college athlete." Instead, my goals became about my own performance and how I could improve every single day. I reevaluated my lifestyle and my relationships in order to improve my mental health. And I was able to get back to being an athlete in order to alleviate the stress from my medical training, which is pretty hard on the body and mind. When I learned how to carve out some time for me, I fell in love with playing sports again. Through this transformation I did the best thing I could do for my patients: be well myself and embody what I preach.

While completing this second fellowship, my mentor E. Lee Rice, DO, FAOASM, FAAFP, FACSM, and I, along with a few non-physicians, launched the Lifewellness Institute in San Diego. Lee is one of the pioneering doctors of both sports medicine and wellness, and created corporate wellness programs that have been used across the country. Our practice focused on executive health physicals, exercise and nutrition programs, and concierge medicine. Many of our clients were corporate executives, their families, and elite athletes, all of whom were able to increase their performance as a result of achieving true wellness. We found that if our athletes followed the same guidelines we gave our corporate patients (who are typically interested in longevity, anti-aging, and heart health), their performance improved.

Every day, new research confirms that physical exercise is a highly effective way of treating and preventing the main causes of aging. We found that we can turn this equation on its head, and use lifestyle enhancements to increase performance, without resorting to growth hormone or other hormonal performance enhancing therapies. Instead, by improving nutrition and sleep, lowering internal toxicity, enhancing exercise recovery and fatigue prevention, as well as developing healthy relationships, our athletes excelled. What's more, by providing the right types of exercise that complement individual training, we learned how to prevent many of the most common problems athletes face in the long run, including ankle, knee, shoulder, and lower back injuries.

Although I loved working with Lee and the team, after ten years it was time to move back to the East Coast to be closer to my family. I joined a sports medicine practice started by my senior resident in family medicine, Clifford Stark, DO, called Sports Medicine at Chelsea in New York City. I started to think about how I could tailor a new wellness protocol based on my own unique view. Today, I use the Step Up Your Game approach for every patient, even for something as minor as a cold. I teach my patients that they are the owner of their health, and by providing them with this framework, they have a tangible way to take care of themselves.

First, we identify where they are at in terms of addressing the nine core categories. I have them visualize each of the nine roles, just like you will learn how to do, so that they can see where the holes are in their own total health program. Then together, we figure out how the nine roles can be implemented.

While I've had lots of success using this program with my "average" patients, I've found that the athletes I work with benefit the most. Athletes respond because they already have a commitment in their minds to achieve change. According to James O. Prochaska, author of *Changing for Good*, people who successfully change their behavior go through a series of five stages, and those who are most successful are able to match their goals to their stage of change. These include *pre-contemplation*, which is the resistance to change, *contemplation* or the acknowledgment of a problem and a search for a solution; *preparation*, the planning stage; and *action*, where the modification of behaviors begins. Finally, the *maintenance* stage allows them to consolidate the gains made in the action stage and work to prevent relapses. More often than not, the athletes who come to see me are at least in the preparation stage. However, I've found that one of the secret successes of my program is its ability to move anyone from contemplation to action as quickly as possible. If you've read this far, you are ready for making the changes necessary to step up your game.

The Sports Grid

The following chart, which I call the Sports Grid, is the core resource for beginning this program. This grid is based on the landmark "Classification of Sport" article all sports medicine physicians are taught to commit to memory. In fact, I was taught during my sports medicine fellowship by one of the authors, Dr. Steven Van Camp, a cardiologist who served as president of the American College of Sports Medicine from 1995 to 1996. It was first created in 1985 and most recently updated by the American College of Cardiology Foundation in 2005 at the 36th Bethesda Conference as a way to classify certain sports to determine whether each was reasonably safe to recommend for an athlete with a specific cardiovascular problem. These researchers organized the sports based on their particular dynamic and static exercise characteristics.

The terms dynamic and static exercise characterize activity on the basis of the action of the muscles involved, but I find that they are analogous for our purposes to the terms most athletes are familiar with: aerobic and anaerobic exercise. They characterize activity on the basis of the type of metabolism the muscles use. Most high-intensity static exercise is performed anaerobically, whereas high-intensity dynamic exercise lasting for more than several minutes is performed aerobically. Some dynamic exercises, such as sprinting or jumping, are performed primarily anaerobically. Whether you are a beginner, intermediate, or performing at the expert level, your chosen sport is most often a mixture of aerobic and anaerobic activity.

For our purposes, I have modified the original chart to include a wider variety of sports, and redefined the parameters. My new grid allows you to quantify your activity based on physical effort. Once you determine where your chosen activity falls, you will be able to personalize your program with the latest nutrition and cross-training recommendations that suit your specific needs. You'll also learn how to analyze your chosen sport and see if you are best suited for it, or if you want to explore other options that might make meeting your fitness goals easier.

Level I Aerobic	Level II Aerobic	Level III Aerobic	
Sector 1	**Sector 2**	**Sector 3**	**Level III Anaerobic**
• Arm-Wrestling • Bobsledding • Cheerleading • Climbing • Dance Team • Field Events (Throwing) • Gymnastics • Judo • Karate • Krav Maga • Luge • Sailing • Water Skiing • Weight Lifting • Windsurfing	• Ballroom Dance • Body Building • Cycling–BMX • Downhill Skiing • Mountain Biking • Skateboarding • Snowboarding • Wrestling	• Boxing • Canoeing • CrossFit • Kayaking • Rowing • Speed (Track) Cycling • Speed Skating • Stair Climbing • Triathlon • Water Polo	
Sector 4	**Sector 5**	**Sector 6**	**Level II Anaerobic**
• Archery • Auto Racing • BASE Jumping • Diving • Equestrian • Fly Fishing • Hang Gliding • Motocross	• Dodgeball • Figure Skating • Football • Field Events (Jumping) • Obstacle Racing • Parkour • Paintball • Rugby • Running (Speed-sprint) • Surfing • Synchronized Swimming	• Basketball • Cross-country skiing (skating technique) • Road Cycling • Ice Hockey • Lacrosse • Paddle boarding • Running (5K To 10K) • Street/Roller Hockey • Swimming • Team Handball	

Level I Aerobic	Level II Aerobic	Level III Aerobic	
Sector 7	Sector 8	Sector 9	Level I Anaerobic
• Bocce Ball • Bowling • Cricket • Darts • Golf • Riflery • Scuba Diving • Shuffleboard • Skeet Shootings	• Baseball • Fencing • Hiking • Softball • Table Tennis • T-Ball • Volleyball	• Badminton • Cross-country Skiing (Classic Technique) • Field hockey • Handball • Inline skating • Orienteering • Race walking • Racquetball • Running (Long Distance) • Soccer • Squash • Tennis • Ultimate Frisbee	

How This Book Works

If there's one thing I know, it's that there's an overabundance of information out there that's supposed to improve your performance. Sometimes I think that's what the Internet was created for! Yet this bombardment of information can do more harm than good. Some websites promote really harmful substances or practices. How are we supposed to separate the wheat from the chaff?

My goal, first and foremost, is to help you systematically understand the best practices of each of the nine roles, provide the most professional information based on actual science, and remove the uncertainty and stress that can occur when you get bogged down in the minutiae of opinions or in false information. You can be assured that I've done the heavy lifting for you; culling through all of the latest research and presenting it in a way so that you can keep focusing on your goals. This will simplify your training, and you'll feel supported by the knowledge that everything you need to succeed can be found in this one book. Then, when life throws you a curveball that results in injury or setbacks, you will already have the resources lined up so that you can immediately get back in the game.

This book addresses both the physical and psychological components to attaining peak performance, along with injury prevention, a comprehensive nutrition program, workouts that support any athletic endeavor, and an overall wellness plan by identifying how each of the nine roles plays a part. Its holistic approach also focuses on the importance of spiritual growth and moral integrity, on and off the field. You will meet some of the leaders in these fields, and learn firsthand their tools and tricks which are guaranteed to get results. What's more, you'll also meet some of the world's elite athletes, and learn how these roles have contributed to their success. Contributors include:

- Adam Krikorian: 2012 US Olympic Committee National Coach of the Year, 2012 Olympic Gold Medal coach, USA Women's Water Polo
- Dean Reinmuth: Professional golf coach for Ricky Barnes and Phil Mickelson (early in his career)
- Ed White: Former NFL football player, College Hall of Fame, San Diego Charger Hall of Fame
- Elizabeth Armstrong: 2012 Olympic Gold Medalist, USA Women's Water Polo
- Heather Fuhr: Professional triathlete, 1997 IRONMAN World Champion, fifteen-time IRONMAN Champion
- Joe Hippensteel: Physical therapist for professional baseball players, Navy SEALS, and Olympians, former national level decathlete

- Peter Holmberg: Olympic silver medalist, sailing, and America's Cup winner in 2007
- Burt Giges, MD: Past president Association for Applied Sport Psychology; Special consultant for USA Track and Field
- Roch Frey: Former professional triathlete, coach for 1997 IRONMAN Hawaii Champion Heather Fuhr and 1998 and 2000 IRONMAN Hawaii Champion Peter Reid
- Shawn Hueglin: Senior sport dietitian, United States Olympic Committee
- Tony Azevedo: Four time Olympian and 2008, 2012 Captain USA Men's Water Polo
- Tucker Dupree: 2012 Paralympian silver medalist, Swimming
- Wendy Hilliard: Former National Team Rhythmic Gymnast, Inductee, USA Gymnastics Hall of Fame, president of Women's Sports Foundation

Now, It's Your Turn

It's very likely that you have already put a lot of work into your chosen sport. That effort may be paying off, or you might need some assistance getting to the next level. Let me help get you there, simply by teaching you how to allocate your resources—your talent, skill, and focus—to put you in the best position to reach your ultimate goal. That's the battle.

The good news is that the journey is going to be fun. We will create the ultimate support system that will meet your specific physical and mental needs. Together we can fine-tune your game, sharpen strengths and attack weaknesses. Best of all, you'll be able to implement a thoughtful plan, just like elite athletes use, that takes into account your daily, weekly, monthly, and yearly needs.

In the next chapter, you'll take the first step toward greatness. We'll define what your short- and long-term goals are by creating your unique athletic mission statement. Then, you'll take a simple quiz to see if you are already addressing any of these roles, and how you can improve on your existing program. You will discover which roles are missing from your training regimen, and how all of the roles fit together in a unique way. Then, you'll be able to fill in your deficient areas as you learn from the experts in their field. Let's get started.

CHAPTER 1
CREATING A PLAYBOOK: DETERMINING GOALS, STRENGTHS, AND DEFICIENCIES

If you aren't going all the way, why go at all?
—*Joe Namath*

Elite athletes succeed because they follow a plan; let's call it their playbook. The playbook holds lots of specific information about their sport: the rules, game day tactics, a workout schedule, and important training information which might include a nutrition plan and inspirational guidance. When elite athletes use their playbook they are taking ownership of their training. This careful planning allows them to not only reach the next level of success, but make good decisions along the way.

Think of this book as your playbook. Each of the nine roles in the elite athlete entourage will provide the same information elite athletes have at their disposal. By understanding the domains and responsibilities these roles take on, and how they interconnect, you can develop an individualized program that will build on your strengths and correct your weaknesses. And by following their suggestions, you'll see real improvements, not only in terms of your athletic performance, but in every facet of your health.

A playbook typically opens with two core ideas: where an athlete wants to go with their skills, and a roadmap for how to get there. Elite athletes are typically goal oriented. They visualize the finish line, the medal, or how it will feel when they realize their dream. Your goals should express what you want to accomplish, whether it's trying a new sport or taking your game to the next level.

You're reading this book because you may already have a specific athletic aspiration you'd like to achieve. Or, you might want to learn how to be the best at your sport, or play at your best without incurring injury. Your motivation may come from rekindling an old yearning from youth, being corralled by a group of friends, or just the innate need to get healthy. Regardless of your intentions, if you use the tools of the playbook, you will be able to achieve your aspiration in an organized and safe way.

Your goals will be created from these aspirations. Ultimately, they have to be distinctive, yet they can be broad or specific, quantifiable or qualitative. Their range depends on where you are in terms of athleticism. No matter what you want to achieve, all goals are valid, including:

- To be more physically fit or more healthy
- To join a gym
- To work out more often and on a regular schedule
- To improve your tennis game and be ranked a 3.5 instead of a 3.0
- To run an eight-minute mile
- To make a high school/college varsity team
- To win a gold medal at the Olympics

We can start to fill in your playbook by parsing out your real goals from your current aspirations: identifying exactly what you want to achieve in both long-term and short-term increments. This exercise falls into two parts: first, creating an overarching athletic mission statement, then defining your specific goals. Together, these strategies will provide the necessary guidance for your journey toward athletic excellence.

The Athletic Mission Statement

Whether your particular aspiration is big or small, you first need to recognize why you want to accomplish it and how you envision yourself achieving it. The tool elite athletes use for uncovering this information is creating a mission statement. Your goals are the momentary steps that will change as you progress, but your mission statement is your greatest motivation, and forms the basis of how you want to live your life on and off the field.

Everyone has a particular mission in life, whether they know it or not. Those who do not fully realize this are less likely to achieve their specific goals. That's because when you are fully aware of your mission, it's easier to get passionate about achieving your goals, which is the greatest internal motivator. And when you're highly motivated, you may find that your performance becomes natural and effortless, which is the secret to ensuring athletic success.

Creating a mission statement helps to solidify your mission by reflecting back your core values. It can identify the underlying causes of behaviors, as well as motivate you to create behavioral change. As Stephen Covey wrote in *The 7 Habits of Highly Effective People*, a mission statement "defines the personal, moral, and ethical guidelines within which you can most happily express and fulfill yourself." In terms of athletics, I believe that a mission statement answers the question, "How can I reveal my true potential?"

Some elite athletes use their mission statement as their mantra, and find that it is one of their best motivators. I teach this skill to my athletic patients in order to help them refocus their goals and priorities, and identify the obstacles that may be blocking their path. What's more, I've found that when they can tell others about their intentions by sharing their mission statement, they are more likely to succeed. This is particularly true when they tell their entourage. By doing so, they ensure that everyone who is managing their training is literally on the same page.

A mission statement is very personal; it is your reason for being, and probably the underlying thoughts that drew you to this book in the first place. Determining it requires a bit of self-exploration and acceptance as well as an opportunity to create new dreams and possibilities. It also gives you a moral grounding so that when you are faced with challenges, you can overcome them. Every decision you make is either consistent with your mission statement and goals, or is not. For example, if your mission statement is *"I want to be my healthiest self,"* you can measure every meal next to your mission statement. If you choose to booze it up before a competition, that's your choice, but it's not consistent with your mission statement. And when your friends want to go to the "all you can eat" buffet you can use your mission statement to guide you toward making better food choices.

Exercise #1: Creating an Elite Athlete's Mission Statement

We can begin the process of creating a mission statement by clearing the mind of all other extraneous thoughts. I like to have my patients do a little meditating for ten minutes or so, or just some deep breathing. There are many ways to meditate, and if you ask twenty people who know how to meditate for instructions, you likely will get twenty different answers. It does not need to be complicated: Find a comfortable place where you can be alone. Turn off all technology. Some athletes like to meditate on their game field. For example, you may choose to sit at the tennis court, walk along a track or your running route, or simply be at home.

The following meditation exercise will help you pinpoint what your mission statement should include:

1. *Meditative breathing*—Breathe in through your nose, then out through your mouth. Feel your abdomen rise with every inhalation. The exhalation should be without effort. Continue to breathe this way for two minutes. You should start to become more relaxed. Let the mind go as you concentrate on your

breathing for the next eight minutes. Feel the sensation of deep relaxation, and do not worry about remembering anything that pops into and out of your head.

2. *Visualization*—In your mind's eye form a mental picture of what the ideal outcome looks like when you are achieving your goals. It may be crossing the finish line, shaking hands with your opponents on the field, or getting a medal on the podium. Fill in as many details as possible. If you have difficulty creating your own mental picture, find one in a magazine or on the Internet that inspires you. Hold that image in your hand, or in your mind, for two full minutes.

3. *Interpretation*—Quickly, write down the first thirty words that come to mind that are related to your chosen sport in the grid below. Don't think too much about them; just write the words down. These thirty words are an investigation into your aspirations. Within this list it's very likely to find some words that are representative of your goals, but you could be surprised by some of the words that surface. Remember, there are no wrong answers! Cross out any negative words that come up. While they are important to get off your chest, they won't serve you well moving forward. Then, circle the words that most closely match your goals.

Aspirational Words

1.	2.	3.	4.	5.
6.	7.	8.	9.	10.
11.	12.	13.	14.	15.
16.	17.	18.	19.	20.
21.	22.	23.	24.	25.
26.	27.	28.	29.	30.

Following the meditation exercise, the next step is to uncover your core values. These are the ideals that you can't live without that are specific to your athletic pursuits. They can be descriptive words of how your sport makes you feel. Or it can be the ideal that you are working toward achieving. It could be self-love. It could be feeling connected, it could be your love for being part of a team.

Review the following list and circle the five words that best describe your core values:

Accomplishment	Generous	Nurturing
Achieving	Genuine	Obedient
Action-oriented	Good	Objective
Appreciation	Gracious	Openness
Ardent	Grateful	Opportunity
Belief	Happy	Optimistic
Careful	Helpful	Organization
Caring	Honest	Original
Clean	Honorable	Outstanding
Credible	Hope	Performance
Daring	Imagination	Perseverance
Dedicated	Integrity	Persistent
Dependable	Intelligence	Planning
Determined	Joyful	Professionalism
Durable	Kindness	Resourceful
Energetic	Knowledge	Stability
Enthusiastic	Lasting	Strength
Ethical	Learning	Sturdy
Equality	Legacy	Togetherness
Excellence	Love	Tough
Faithful	Malleable	Truth
Fearless	Mastery	Unity
Finesse	Meaningful	Valiant
Forgiveness	Memorable	Vigorous
Formidable	Nimble	Wisdom
Free-thinking	Noble	Youthful
Fun	Novel	Zen

Then, record your five core values:

1.

_____

2.

_____

3.

_____

4.

_____

5.

_____

With your core values and your aspirational words in mind, write down the answers to the following questions:

How do you want to be remembered?

_____

What matters most to you?

_____

What are your family's values?

_____

How would you define success?

_____

What does happiness feel like when you are playing your chosen sport?

_____

What would your friends, spouse, or partner say about your athletic venture?

_____

What would your children say about your athletic venture?

_____

If you were thirty years older, what would you say to your present day self?

_____

Next, write three successes you've already achieved in your sport, as well as three failures. This part of the exercise will help you remember the highs and the lows of your athletic career, and how you much you have already endured to get to where you are today.

If you are thinking about transitioning from one sport to another, or have never played a sport and want to start playing one, envision being in that sport and imagine three successes and failures, or think about a star in that sport and research their three biggest successes and failures.

Successes
1.

_____

2.

_____

3.

_____

Failures
1.

_____

2.

_____

3.

_____

Your mission statement is why you're striving toward your goals, doing the hard work. Review your aspirational words, your core values, the answers to the reflective questions, your previous successes and failures. Is there an overall theme? What is the underlying motivation? The answer to this question becomes your personal athletic mission statement. The last step is to distill your athletic mission statement into no more than fifteen words. Memorize it; own it. Whenever you get down, remember your mission statement, and remind yourself why you are invested in your chosen sport. This process may take a few days, some a few weeks. Take whatever time you need: it is vitally important to be completely honest and not rush it.

Some of the most common mission statements I've heard include:

- "To be healthy"
- "To get back to what I enjoy"
- "To explore my athletic potential"

My Athletic Mission Statement: _____

Meet Michael

Michael is a twenty-five-year-old stock broker who ran cross country in college. He has been working hard at building his career since graduating, and he came to see me because he wanted to start running again. He wants to get back into shape, and he's motivated by his girlfriend, Lisa, who also runs and wants to find an activity they can do together.

Michael and I sat down for a consultation. We decided to go through the entire mission statement exercise. After ten minutes of meditation, he wrote down the following and quickly edited out the negative words:

Aspirational Words

Healthy	Breathing	Alive	Heart	Love
Fulfill	Fun	Winning	~~Soreness~~	~~Knee pain~~
Water	Sunny	Outside	Together	Finish
~~Nervous~~	~~Blisters~~	~~Vomit~~	~~Music~~	~~Sweat~~
~~Falling~~	Crowds	Group	Inspire	Pleasure
Finish Line	Race	Friends	Companionship	Morning

<u>Five Core Values</u>

1. Joyful
2. Durable
3. Togetherness
4. Performance
5. Lasting

Michael then answered the reflective questions:

- I want to be remembered for running with a smile.
- Running with my girlfriend is important to me because it would add another positive dimension to our relationship.
- My family values have always been about being athletic.
- Success to me means to run as many races as I can and have fun.
- I was always happy when I was running as a kid.
- My girlfriend believes that running is in me.
- When I have children, I want them to think, "Dad is a great runner!"
- Keep running for fun and with passion, and do not run hurt!

<u>Three Successes:</u>

- Made the varsity team in high school in the tenth grade
- Beat rival in college
- Made captain of team in college

Three Failures:
- Missed making regionals in high school
- Disqualified a few times for false starts
- Overtrained senior year and got injured and missed last half of season

Using these data, Michael and I came up with the following:

Michael's Athletic Mission Statement: *to cross each finish line with joy and a sense of togetherness.*

Setting the Right Goals

The goal-setting process can help athletes understand their current level of mastery and where they want to go. There are two types of goals: subjective and objective. Subjective goals are not related to a specific improvement of skills, but correlated to trying one's best. Objective goals are performance-based and can help athletes focus and improve technical and tactical skills. For example, an objective goal is decreasing time in a swimming event.

Goals should be focused on process and performance during practice rather than on the outcome of any particular competition. Focusing on process and performance-based goals will lead to less anxiety compared to outcomes-based goals (i.e. winning). The more you focus on process goals, the less you will worry about how you perform during competition, and then hopefully will perform better. What's more, these are the types of goals you can have control over, particularly if you play a team sport, where the outcome of a particular game might have nothing to do with you, and everything to do with another player.

SMART Goals Lead to Smart Choices

One goal setting technique I've borrowed from the corporate world and the International Olympic Committee—which has been endorsed by various sport psychologists—is the idea of developing SMART goals. Most athletes do not set SMART goals, but elite athletes do. These goals are defined by their characteristics:

- **Specific**—a goal that targets a single area for improvement, such as achieving a thirty-inch vertical leap from a twenty-five-inch vertical leap, or making a competitive travel team.
- **Measurable**—quantify or at least suggest an indicator of progress, such as improving your timing or your endurance.
- **Attainable**—goals that are neither out of reach nor below your current level of performance. Your goal should also be *adjustable*: once achieved, the next level should be obvious. You can continually reevaluate your goals to see if they change as they are tested with both successes as well as the various stressors in life.
- **Relevant**—goals should be consistent with your mission statement.
- **Timely**—specify how you can commit to this goal by approximating when the result can be achieved.

The advantage of SMART goals is that they are both easy to quantify and easy to recognize when you have achieved them. SMART goals can also be correlated to the other qualities of goal setting. They can be performance-based (achieving a batting average of 300), process-based (having great form at the plate when hitting in baseball) or outcome-based (i.e. winning). Again, focusing on the process- and performance-based goal setting is preferred to the outcome-based. Winning comes more often than not when you are focused on the process and performance.

Let's get back to Michael. His girlfriend had already signed up for a local 5K charity run that was slated to take place three months later. We decided that training for this race would feature performance and process goals. His performance goal would be to focus on keeping his pace at seven minutes per mile. His process goal was to focus on his form. Then, using the SMART goal-setting technique we reviewed the parameters:

- **Specific:** Participate and train for a 5K run.
- **Measurable:** By joining a local team for training and using a fitness tracker, Michael would be able to measure his training progress.
- **Achievable:** 5K is achievable with three months of training. If he wanted to run a marathon in the same amount of time that would not be safely achievable.
- **Relevant:** Training and participating in the race is consistent with his mission statement: *to cross each finish line with joy and a sense of togetherness.*
- **Timely:** Parameters created by the date of race and local team's training schedule.

Exercise #2: Target Specific Goals

Let's revisit your aspirations and compare them to your mission statement in order to create your goals. Your new goals will be the actions required to fulfill the mission. Ask yourself, *"What do your goals mean to you?"*

For example, let's say my objective has been to run a sub-four minute mile. When I ask myself why I am pursuing this and compare it to my athletic mission statement—*to reach my full athletic potential and avoid injury*—I can clearly see a disconnect, because I couldn't run this fast without injuring myself due to my heavier, muscular physical stature. Knowing this I can then outline specific goals that will help me reach a different, more attainable goal of running a sub–six minute mile.

The next step is to determine how you came to your original objective. When I'm working with my athletic patients, I ask them about what motivates them, why it is important to them, what their previous experiences or attempts have been in relation to that goal. There are times when I find the motivation is internal and coming from a pure place. Other times the motivation is external: it can be for fame, to impress another person, or live up to their parents' expectations. I've found that internal motivations typically lead to better results and overall feelings of satisfaction. For example, over the years I've met countless athletes of every level, and every age, who are following the hopes and dreams of their parents, girlfriends or boyfriends, or another important person in their lives, instead of their own. Unless your goals come from your own desires, you will always have difficulty fulfilling them, or worse, develop animosity toward them. This tension is probably the most common cause of hindering ones' true potential. If you know deep down that you are working toward a goal that's not your own, and you're not really excited or passionate about it, then maybe it's time to start thinking about what you can do with your talents that will inspire you. It's never too late to try something new.

Next, let's make sure that the goals you are envisioning are realistic and achievable. Achievable goals tend to be those that can be reached with a clear vision. For example, if a ten-year-old athlete tells me that she wants to be an Olympic softball player, her goal is only realistic and achievable if many other smaller goals can be realized first (i.e. join a local club team, make the junior Olympic or national squad, etc.). In contrast, unachievable and unrealistic goals are not well thought out, and can keep an athlete in a state of disillusionment. For example, I've had patients tell me that they want to run a marathon in the next three months who have never run a mile. I've also worked with boxers who have fought at a certain weight yet are asked to fight in two to three weeks at a weight class higher. Both of these goals are not only unrealistic, they set the athlete up for failure and a high chance for injury.

This is not to say you that you should limit your dreams. In fact, I find too many people don't strive big enough in terms of their athletic hopes. I often wish my patients had more far-fetched, out-of-the-box goals. For example, let's say your goal is to score eight times in a game. First, decide if that goal is realistic based on your skill level. Even if it seems untenable, see if you can create a plan for accomplishing it. Your first goal can be to ensure that you are strong enough or have the talent to score once. The second goal could be to work on your stamina so that you can score a second time, and so on. As you tick off smaller goals, your highest goal will become less of a pipe dream and more of a reality. And then when you meet that ultimate goal, it will be time to set a new one.

By setting big, long-term goals that can be met by breaking them down into small, short-term goals you can tick off successfully, you can focus on the short term and the long term at the same time. Let's say your goal is to run an eight-minute mile. Think for a moment: is that really all you want? Have you considered running a 5K? If so, what would you need to get from where you are now to achieving that bigger goal? Can you set up smaller goals to meet that ultimate goal, such as creating intermediary benchmarks and participating in races in order to qualify? Is it consistent with your athletic mission statement?

As you discover your smaller goals, you might find that the big goal can change with the clarity that is gained. For example, let's say Johnny wants to make a varsity basketball team in high school. He is in the ninth grade and has only been playing pickup basketball. He played freshman ball but did not make the JV team. He has next year to make the JV team, then hopefully make the varsity team in his junior year. That idea of striving to make the varsity basketball team is a motivator, but in order to reach that in another year he still has to create a number of smaller, additional goals. First, he needs to play summer ball to keep his skill fresh. He could attend one or two weekly basketball camps, then try out for JV in the fall.

Now that you have clarified your goals, you're ready to explore the elite athlete's entourage. Each role will provide you with the necessary information to fill out every aspect of your playbook. These roles have been developed to directly support your mission statement and your goals. They are your check-and-balance system. Whenever you feel a conflict with your mission that's when you use that aspect of your entourage. Think of the roles and responsibilities of the entourage as the team that will give you the best chance of living your dream, one that is consistent with your athletic mission statement, and will support your SMART goals.

Meet the Elite Athlete Entourage

Some athletes will address some of the roles of the entourage, but not others. For example, some athletes think cross-training is the key to victory: if they get physically strong that alone will be enough to ensure success. If that doesn't work, they resort to shortcuts like performance enhancers to give them an edge. Yet the elite athlete understands the importance of all of the roles in the entourage, and how they work together, and can make sure all aspects are covered equally in a systematic way.

Let's determine your current strengths and deficiencies, and see how the nine roles of the elite athlete entourage fit in to your existing routine. The nine roles are broken into two groups. The first covers the physical components of training: all the processes and preventive measures you need to think about regarding your body. These roles cover pregame, off-the-field activities that will help improve your field performance: they encompass everything you need to do to get ready to play your best. They are also necessary during and after the game (i.e. a team physician will be available if you get hurt or will develop the game plan to get you back on the field after an injury). Once these processes are put in place, we can start working on the second group, which covers your emotional, mental needs that influence both pregame training and competition.

I have placed these roles in a specific sequential order. As with any new exercise program, you're going to want to see your doctor before you begin. Then, your doctor will work with you to evaluate the rest of the roles as you introduce them into your athletic life.

Group 1: The Physical Roles

The Team Physician: The team physician is your pre-season quarterback. He or she makes sure you're ready to take the field in the best health possible. They also act as the liaison, the *consiglieri*, to each of the other roles. The team physician is not a role that you can take on yourself. However, in the next chapter you'll explore how to work with your own physician to make sure that you are in the best health for your sport.

The Physical Therapist: A physical therapist identifies physical issues that might weaken your ability to play at your highest level. They help you develop physical stability which is needed to build strength and endurance. For example, shoulder pain often occurs as a result of poor posture, and a physical therapist can help you correct your stance as well as provide the necessary stretching to make you more comfortable. The responsibilities of this role can easily be taken on by any athlete. No matter what sport you choose, make sure you engage in the preventative, "pre-hab" exercises featured in Chapter 3 in order to keep you injury free.

The Trainer: A trainer creates and supervises training workouts. They maintain thorough and accurate records, teach proper technique, and create preventive and corrective exercises specific to your sport. The responsibilities of this role can easily be taken on by any athlete. In fact, by assuming this role, your training will become more efficient as well as more effective. The information in Chapter 4 is directly correlated to your sport of choice based on the Sports Grid and will feature both anaerobic and aerobic workouts that align with your unique athletic goals.

The Dietitian: A dietitian makes sure you are adequately nourishing your body in order to optimally support brain function, body function, and recovery from injury. The responsibilities of this role can easily be taken on by any athlete. In Chapter 5, you'll find a week's worth of nutritional guidance that is directly correlated to your sport of choice based on the Sports Grid.

Group 2: The Mental Game

The Coach: The coach is the person you entrust to provide guidance in order for you to give it your all. The coach's role takes place during your activity. He or she ensures that you are prepared for the actual task. The responsibilities of this role can easily be taken on by any athlete. In Chapter 6, you'll find best practices from an individual as well as a team coach, and other resources that will allow you to take on the toughest competitor.

The Competitor: Athletes face lots of competitors, including themselves. When utilized properly, competition can propel you to new heights. In Chapter 7, you'll learn how to identify your primary competitors, and use a competitive rivalry to raise your level of play.

The Role Model/Hero: Having a role model is critical for an elite athlete's success. Many of the men and women I've worked with have been able to identify a person in their lives, or in their sport, that epitomizes what they strive to achieve, and has a proven strategy behind their success that can be replicated. In Chapter 8, you'll learn how to find your role model, and how to be one for other athletes.

The Psychologist: A sport psychologist develops mental strategies that enhance performance. I have found that most great athletes can improve their competitive game by working with a psychologist. This is a role that any athlete can take on for themselves by using their tools and techniques as described in Chapter 9. By doing so, when obstacles come up over the course of training or competition, you will be better prepared to handle them.

The Spiritual Leader: Many of the elite athletes I've worked with are open about their spirituality: they feel connected to a power greater than themselves, and show this connection in a various ways. Many believe, as I do, that this connection can help to take your game to the next level. In Chapter 10, you will learn how to find that extra intangible that the greatest athletes talk about.

Time-Out: Tips from the Pros

Elizabeth "Betsey" Armstrong was the 2012 Gold Medal Goalie for USA Water Polo women's team. I asked her which of these nine roles made the greatest difference in her training leading up to the Olympic Games.

Betsey told me, "I had been a dedicated athlete for the past eighteen years, but I was an English Lit major as an undergrad at the University of Michigan. I never focused on math or science or physiology or biology. All of my education about myself, my body, and being an athlete has come from the experts in the field. For example, my physical therapist leading up to the London Olympics was absolutely remarkable. The pre-hab and re-hab strength and conditioning program we had was so informative and adaptive. He really taught me why I needed to do each exercise and what purpose they had. I was then able to use this knowledge in the pool and look for the differences in my body and in my performance as I played."

Connecting the Roles for Peak Performance

You'll learn much more about each of these roles in the following chapters. As you read, you'll see how they connect with one another and form a cohesive set of instructions that will complete your playbook.

In 2011, I was selected to serve as a volunteer physician at the US Olympic Training Center in Colorado Springs, Colorado, an exceptional facility where qualifying Olympic and Paralympic hopefuls have all of the same resources available as my entourage approach. Upon walking into the medical facility I felt like a kid in a candy store. There were state-of-the-art medical imaging machines, along with every physical therapy tool available. From hand therapy's bucket of millet seed to the then brand new Alter-G machine which allows athletes to run on a treadmill with forces less than gravity while they healed from injury, the modalities available truly allowed us all to feel best able to treat any injury. It was a perfect scenario for serving as a team physician.

Better still, I was able to see exactly how my model worked. These athletes all had access to the highest level of expertise which was available when they needed it. This allowed them to stay focused on their sport performance and constantly improving.

The Sport Performance Department at the USOTC is made up of the following divisions that directly correlate with the Step Up Your Game approach.

- **High Performance:** focuses on leadership and coaching; this unit develops plans and allocates resources that will have the most impact on performance
- **Nutrition:** focuses on providing nutritional services, education, and research
- **Sport Psychology:** prepares athletes for competition and develops mental skills necessary for international competition
- **Strength and Conditioning:** like our strength coach/personal trainer, this department designs and implements scientific, sport specific strength and conditioning programs
- **Physiology:** like our physical therapist, this department analyzes different responses to exercise in regard to its effect on cardiovascular and muscle performance and recovery
- **Sports Medicine:** provides comprehensive medical care to the athlete

And of course, the athletes were surrounded with their fiercest competitors, as well as their role models.

The Step Up Your Game Quiz

Now that you can imagine how each of these roles will influence your play and your training, let's see what you are already incorporating into your existing routine. The following questions are meant to inspire self-reflection. You may find that your existing regimen addresses some of the issues related to these roles already, but not in a structured or systematic way.

If you answer "yes" to all four questions within a category, you may very well be proficient in that role and can move on to the next. If you answer "yes" to two or three questions in the category, you are knowledgeable, but may require help beefing up that role. If you answer "yes" to one or none, you need to incorporate more of that role into your training. Regardless of your score, I do recommend reading through each of these roles, if for nothing else than to see if the expert advice matches what you already know.

Team Physician

- Do you research what medical treatments are available for your injuries/illnesses and discuss it with him/her because your physician is well versed in athletic issues?
- Is your physician an athlete?
- Does your physician think holistically in taking care of all aspects of your athletic self (i.e. he or she addresses supplements, overtraining, training errors)?
- Does your physician assimilate all the information you present to her/him and create meaning that pertains to your life/athletic self?

Physical Therapist

- After getting injured, do you immediately stop your sport and rest in order to recover?
- Do you know a core set of exercises that will keep your injury from recurring or keep you injury-free?
- Do you do the necessary exercises that will keep your injury from recurring or keep you injury-free?
- Are you knowledgable regarding the most common injuries related to your sport?

Trainer

- Do you have an understanding of cardio, strength training, and flexibility exercises that can be used for your sport?
- Do you have a good understanding of the type of exercises that will functionally improve your performance in your sport (i.e. overhead weights to improving throwing)?
- Is your speed/strength not improving despite having adequate nutrition?
- Do you find yourself getting hurt when going to work out due to poor form/biomechanics?

Dietitian

- Do you feel your performance is not at its best despite exercising regularly?
- Do you have a plan for changing your eating pattern for different stages of your training for competition (i.e. off-season training, in-season training, pregame, postgame, while traveling)?
- Do you have a hard time managing your energy needs with your expenditure?
- Do you have a hard time gaining muscle despite regular weightlifting/conditioning?

Coach

- Do you consistently hit a wall when trying to increase your performance?
- Do you have the ability to be honest with yourself when trying to play your sport, or do you make excuses when you don't perform to the best of your ability?
- Do you have a hard time keeping with your goals or do you get easily distracted?
- Do you know the ins and outs of your game, from rules to positioning, etc.?

Competitor

- Who are your top three competitors in your sport?
- Do you see yourself as a worthy competitor of others or your best self?
- Do you view the competitor as an enemy that needs to be destroyed, or as a means to raise your game?
- Have you studied the training practices of your competitor?

Role Model/Hero

- Can you quickly remember your childhood idol?
- Do you have a role model/hero you actively follow?
- Are you aware of a role model/hero within your chosen sport?
- Does your idol motivate your passion for your sport?

Psychologist

- Do you have relationship or unresolved personal issues that keep you from performing at your best?
- Do you feel alone or disconnected?
- Are you distracted by life's stresses that keep you from performing at your best?
- Do you have a mental strategy for both pregame and game time?

Spiritual Leader

- Do you feel connected to a community outside of your sport?
- Do you feel that you are a part of something bigger than yourself?
- Do you have a strategy to tap into something other than yourself in order to play to your best abilities?
- Do you have a pregame or postgame meditation practice?

Meet Carrie

My patient Carrie is a thirty-five-year-old mother of two who realized that keeping up with her children was getting increasingly difficult. She married her college sweetheart, who was the captain of the football team, yet Carrie had never considered herself as particularly athletic. During her annual physical, Carries asked if I could advise her as to how she could best get in shape to become a recreational soccer player. Her kids were both on traveling soccer teams and she wanted to understand the game better and get into shape. She also thought it would be a great way to bond with her kids. I told Carrie that her idea was the basis of a strong mission statement, and that I thought her goals were achievable. I then gave her the *Step Up Your Game* quiz to determine her proficiency in the various roles. Of course, she already had me as a team physician, so she scored a 4 on Question 1.

Carrie scored the following:

Team physician: 4
Physical therapist: 2
Personal trainer: 2
Dietitian: 3
Coach: 2
Competitor: 2
Idol: 0
Psychologist: 2
Spiritual Leader: 4

Based upon her scores, we focused on building out her playbook in the following categories: I would act as her physician. For the role of the physical therapist, I gave her some specific stretches to work on that met her soccer goals, as well as a set of pre-hab exercises to prevent back and leg injuries. For the role of dietitian, we discussed the basics of a nutritious diet that would give her enough energy for her new sport. For the role of the trainer, I outlined a cardio and strength-training program that would start after becoming proficient with the pre-hab exercises. For coach, I had her look at a soccer website that gave some basics on the rules of the game as well as a tutorial to learn the mechanics of the most common movements in soccer. For the competitor, she identified herself as her strongest competitor, since she was entirely new to the game. For the psychologist, I gave her some information on visualization techniques that could help her relax when preparing and playing a game. Because she did not grow up playing soccer, she adopted one of her son's idols, Lionel Messi. I asked her to watch a *60 Minutes* segment on Lionel Messi's career so she could learn more about him. Carrie was already the spiritual leader of her family, and enjoyed taking them to church frequently.

We then discussed her goals using the SMART technique:

- **Specific**—I want to play soccer in a pickup league that is going to start in the spring.
- **Measurable**—I will dedicate three times per week for working on my soccer game and general fitness, using the resources provided by Dr. Rao.
- **Attainable**—I am in good health and have put aside the time required, so playing in the league should be attainable.
- **Relevant**—It is in alignment with my athletic mission statement "to be healthy and connected to my children."
- **Timely**—three months is reasonable to get in shape for the upcoming season and to learn the game in order to participate at the beginner level league.

Carrie now had a plan. She felt confident that she had the resources put into place in order for her to get on the soccer field. Knowing that her roles were taken care of, she started following the diet and exercise routines outlined in the next few chapters. And in about eight weeks, she felt like she could keep up with the rest of the women on her recreational team.

The same can be true for you. Once you fully understand the roles that you need to take on, you'll see how every aspect of your training comes together. Like all good fitness programs, you should have a complete physical before you begin. That's why the first role you'll explore is the team physician.

CHAPTER 2
THE TEAM PHYSICIAN

The team physician provides for the well-being of individual athletes, enabling each to realize his/her full potential.

—The American Osteopathic Academy of Sports Medicine

During my residency in family medicine I was introduced to my first mentor in sports medicine, Richard Levandowski, MD. He was and still is the team physician for the Hun School of Princeton in New Jersey as well as other local high schools and small colleges. He also was named the head physician for the Special Olympics 2014 USA Games. On the field Dr. Levandowski was ready to tackle any medical issue that couldn't be handled by the athletic trainer, and made sure emergency planning was in place by establishing a relationship with the onsite ambulance team. I was impressed with both the way he took care of the athletes and how he interacted with the athletic department, and I knew from watching him that his methods were exactly the way I wanted to practice medicine. For example, before a high school football game the star running back came over with a tender, ingrown toe nail that was causing so much pain he couldn't run. Even though it was a minor injury, it was having a big impact on this player's performance.

Dr. Levandowski went into his medical bag and pulled out his scissors, clamps, betadine and gauze, and within ten minutes had the running back up and on the field. The sighs of relief were palpable by the coaching staff and teammates.

Like Dr. Levandowski, all team physicians oversee the total well-being of their athletes. This role encompasses all aspects of play: pregame training, competition, and postgame recovery. Off the field they create a preventive approach to health to avoid illness and injury, and can diagnose existing problems and resolve them either before you start your program or put you on a protocol so that they can be resolved during your program. On the field they are typically the first to recognize and intervene during health-related emergency situations, as well as the major and minor cuts, bumps, and bruises that occur during play. Afterwards, they continue to monitor your health so that you can be at your peak throughout your athletic career.

A team physician is not a job you want to take on yourself. Any athlete, at any level needs a real doctor. In this chapter you'll learn about the team physician's main tasks and how you can make sure your doctor is ensuring that you reach your highest athletic potential.

The Qualities of a Team Physician

Working with the right team physician can form a relationship that lasts a lifetime, so it's important to make sure your current doctor is serving you well. The ideal qualification of a team physician is a Family Medicine practitioner who specializes in Sports Medicine. This means they will have completed a fellowship in Sports Medicine and have passed the certification exam, obtaining a Certificate of Added Qualifications (CAQ). While many other types of doctors can be one's team physician, Family Medicine physicians are trained to see the big picture because they treat a lifetime of health. They also have the ability to synthesize disparate pieces of information to come up with a comprehensive and individualized program. On top of that, a doctor who specializes in Sports Medicine not only understands musculoskeletal injury management but also injury prevention, nutrition, exercise, and psychology.

I believe that an osteopathically trained (DO vs. MD) primary care sports medicine physician is the ideal team physician because DOs practice a "whole person" approach to medicine. Instead of just treating specific symptoms or illnesses, they regard the body as an integrated whole. I have plenty of MD colleagues who also embody the osteopathic philosophy, like Dr. Levandowski. Both DOs and MDs are fully qualified physicians licensed to prescribe medication and perform surgery. DOs receive extra training in the musculoskeletal system—the body's interconnected system of bones, joints, muscles, ligaments, cartilage, and tendons. This training is particularly useful for athletes as it allows the team physician to better understand how an illness or injury in one part of your body can affect other parts. DOs are also qualified to perform Osteopathic Manipulative Treatment, a specific type of hands-on training that can be used to treat and diagnose various illness/injuries. This technique is a valuable tool that can replace the need for medications other traditional treatments in many instances, or it can be used in conjunction with them.

Some of the best team physicians I have had the pleasure of working with are sports chiropractors. These men and women have an in-depth knowledge of sports medicine, and know how to coordinate care for athletes. In fact, one of my colleagues, Bill Moreau, DC, DACBSP, CSCS is a sports chiropractor and the managing director of the US Olympic Committee Sports Medicine Division. Sports chiropractors have a comprehensive approach to the care of the athlete, and with the help of a medical doctor (DO or MD), who can prescribe medications and perform procedures like injections and surgery, can provide the care you may need.

One of the most important tasks for a team physician is to guide athletes to make decisions that support their unique requirements for performance. Working with a right-brained, creative team physician is key for arriving at medically sound decisions. The right-brained physician uses intuition, feeling, and artfulness in order to make sense of the limitless data, interpret it in a meaningful way, and apply it to your individual needs. A good team physician will take into account every injury in the context of the athlete: how does it affect their psyche? Is it going to affect the team dynamics? For example, an ankle sprain won't mean the same thing for every athlete, and the treatment will change whether you are in preseason training or in the middle of a game.

It's quite likely that you will intuitively realize if your doctor has a right-brained mentality. He or she will be able to communicate well, synthesize multiple aspects of your particular issues, and create a recommendation that is uniquely tailored to your needs instead of using a cookie-cutter approach. If you believe that you're not getting this type of individualized attention, it might be time to look for a new team physician.

10 Questions Every Team Physician Should Be Able to Answer

I have worked with plenty of athletes who want to meet me before their first exam to see if we are the right fit. Here are the top ten questions I suggest you ask:

1. *What are your credentials?* An osteopathic sports medicine doctor who is family medicine–based is the gold standard, but I'm biased to these credentials. The truth is, any doctor who shares this philosophy would be a good choice, such as a primary care physician—certified as either a Family Medicine practitioner, pediatrician (covering birth through age eighteen, some to twenty-one) or an internist—especially if they currently work as a team physician for a local team. Most primary care physicians will be looking at ways to prevent disease, but they may not address performance, which is the skill set you are looking for.

2. *What is your availability?* It's important to know your doctor's office hours, and how they handle crises. They should have regular working hours throughout the week with on-call availability for emergencies that occur on nights and on weekends. Ideally they can work with other doctors you can meet to create 24/7 coverage.

3. *What kind of role will you take in my care?* Your doctor can tell you if they are more of a disease-based or preventive-based practitioner.

Look for one who takes a preventive approach that can coordinate care within your health care system.

4. *Are you well versed in the ailments that are common to my athletic pursuits?* A true team physician knows how to treat patients based upon their unique circumstances, and be well aware of "in season" vs "out of season" management of injury/illness. For example, if you are a tennis player, you don't necessarily need a doctor who is a tennis player, or even one who treats other tennis players. However, the doctor does need to be familiar with the various ailments that may be common for those who play tennis, such as calf strains.

5. *What hospital are you affiliated with?* In order to affiliate with a hospital, doctors must go through a stringent review process, which is one of the reasons why the best doctors are always affiliated. Hospital networks also provide increased access to care, so this question addresses the additional resources you will be able to tap into in terms of continuity of care. A good physician will have access to the right medical technology and is a part of a network of specialists.

6. *How much time would you spend with me for a typical office visit?* The right answer should be, "That depends." Your doctor may be able to resolve your issue in as little as five minutes, or may require thirty minutes or more to resolve complex issues, but it's not the amount of time spent with you that really matters. Instead, I believe the quality of the time that they spend with you is far more important. I've seen plenty of doctors staring at their smartphone when they should be engaged with their patients. Your doctor should give you 100 percent of his or her attention: they should look you in the eye and give you the presence you deserve.

7. *How is your front office run?* I can judge a doctor by how well they run their front office. Is the staff welcoming? Is the office neat? If the front office knows what they're doing, it shows me that the

doctors are putting time and effort into their staff, which means they'll put the time and effort into your treatment plan too.

8. *Are you an athlete?* Your doctor should be an athlete, or at least someone who embodies wellness. This is important because being athletic embodies a wellness philosophy. Go to their website and look at the physician's profile, and you'll see what their activities and hobbies are. Every team physician doesn't have to be a marathon runner or a triathlete, but they should have some sporty interest that they're willing to highlight in their profile.

9. *What are your typical "return to play" guidelines?* Many doctors tell athletes to stop working out entirely for a week or even a month after an injury when there is no evidence to support that recommendation. The truth is there are many ways to keep one going. While doctors are instructed to "do no harm," a true team physician will know how to keep you active even when you are injured, if possible. With all of the current rehabilitation modalities, the circumstances are far and few between when I absolutely say one should not be active when recovering from an injury. There are many circumstances that will require an athlete to stop training, and a good team physician can help them cross train in another way while dealing with that injury.

10. *Are you open to learning new information?* Team physicians should be up to date with the current research, or have the resources available if needed. It's quite likely that your existing doctor may not have all of these qualifications, but as long as he or she is open to learning more about your particular pursuit and the care you might require, or can refer you to someone who meets your specific needs as they come up, you should be fine.

The Step Up Your Game Sports Physical

Once you find a doctor that you like and trust, schedule a physical where you can discuss your athletic goals. Your physician will be diagnosing existing problems and resolving them either before you start this program or as you continue through. Aside from making sure that you are healthy enough to expend energy, he or she will also want to create a set of baseline reference points to be able to track progress.

Every physical will be slightly different, depending on your age, gender, and risk factors for diseases. The following questionnaire lists the components of a typical sports medicine physical that your doctor can modify to meet your specific needs. It's always a good idea to keep your own personal health records including lab results, imaging results, consultation reports, etc. If you don't know the answers to all of these questions now, your doctor can help you fill in the data after your physical.

Step Up Your Game Health Questionnaire	
QUESTIONS	RECORD YOUR ANSWERS HERE
Date	
Name	
Date of Birth	
Health Professional Contact List	List all health professionals you currently see: doctors, trainers, dieticians, psychologists, etc.:
Heath Care Records Review	List any records/testing results from previous or current health care professionals (attach records if available):
List Goals and Concerns	Include your goals from Chapter 1:

Past Medical History	List known medical conditions as well as current or past injuries/illnesses:
Pre-Participation Exam	Answer the following yes or no: Exertional chest pain or discomfort, or shortness of breath? Have you ever passed out or felt like you were going to pass out after exercise? (exertional syncope or near-syncope) Past detection of cardiac murmur or systemic hypertension? Known family history of hypertrophic cardiomyopathy—(abnormally thickened heart, other cardiomyopathies, long QT syndrome (abnormal electrical heart disease), Marfan syndrome (genetic disorder of connective tissue), or significant dysrhythmias (abnormal electrical heart diseases)? Family history of premature death or known disabling cardiovascular disease in close family relative younger than fifty years?
Past Surgical History	List any surgeries:
Allergies	Include medications, food, environmental, etc.:

Alternative Medicine List	List complementary/alternative therapies you participate in, such as Acupuncture, Rolfing, Ayurvedic medicine:
Family History	List diseases/causes of the family members, including parents, siblings, and grandparents:
Concussion History	List individual occurrences and approximate time it took for complete recovery:
Eating Disorder History	Have you ever been diagnosed with an eating disorder?
Depression Screening	Do you have little interest or pleasure in doing things? Do you feel down, depressed, or hopeless?
Medications	List all medications you have recently taken or are currently taking:

Supplements	List all supplements you have recently taken or are currently taking:
Tobacco Use and History	Include smoking, chewing; include frequency and if you use now or have used in the past:
Alcohol History	List how many alcoholic drinks per week:
Drugs	Include illicit and performance-enhancing; include frequency and if you use now or have used in the past:
Nutrition	Record a typical one day food diary, including all meals, snacks, and beverages: Breakfast: Lunch: Dinner: Snack(s): Beverages:

Exercise	Record a week's worth of exercise history in minutes and times per week: Aerobic: Weights/Resistance Training: Team Sports: Stretching:
Stress	On a scale of 1–10, how do you rate your stress level (1 being little stress, 10 being high stress):
Spirituality	On a scale of 1–10, how do you rate your sense of spirituality (1 being low and 10 being high):

Testing Your Doctor Should Recommend

Your team physician should teach you about your numbers, risk for disease/injury, and develop a solid wellness plan that is consistent with your goals.

- Vitals: weight, height, BMI (body mass index), waist circumference, heart rate, blood pressure (risk factor for heart disease)
- Orthopedic screening exam: check for joint issues
- Visual acuity: check for visual defects that are >20/40
- Basic lipid panel: tests for risk of heart disease (cholesterol, LDL, HDL, and triglycerides)

- Comprehensive metabolic panel: tests for diabetes, electrolytes, liver and kidney function
- TSH (thyroid stimulating hormone): test for thyroid health
- Urinalysis: test for bladder or kidney issues and screens for certain metabolic disorders
- CBC (complete blood count check): for infection, anemia, and platelet disorders
- B12 (for vegetarians): vitamin important for red blood cell production
- Vitamin D: vitamin important for bone health
- Ferritin: measure of iron storage
- Electrocardiogram (if any cardiac risk factors): tests for cardiac abnormalities
- Exercise stress test: the American College of Sports Medicine suggests this for men forty years and older, women fifty years and older, and for athletes engaging in vigorous exercise
- DEXA scan: for bone density and risk for osteoporosis
- Immunizations: refer to immunization schedule at www.cdc.gov/vaccines/schedules/

Critical Conversations to Have with Your Doctor

When you work with a team physician you are forming a relationship. And like any good partnership, it depends on transparency. I cannot stress enough the importance of having an honest relationship with your doctor. It's like the techies say, "garbage in, garbage out." The output—how well your doctor manages your health—is directly related to the information you provide. If your doctor does not have all the pertinent information regarding your health, he or she will not be an asset to your entourage, and will not be able to successfully coordinate the other roles. Simply put, the whole Step Up Your Game program hinges on your honest relationship with your doctor.

This is particularly important when patients are recovering from previous injuries or taking medications, including prescriptions, over-the-counter remedies, nutraceuticals, performance enhancers, or even recreational drugs. Whatever high-risk behavior you might be participating in needs to be fully discussed. Rest assured, a good team physician won't judge the behavior. The team physician is an adviser, plain and simple, whose role is to be there for the athlete without judgment, to show empathy, and provide medical facts. The days when doctors were viewed as all-knowing parents are over—when the doctor laid down the law, you listened. Today, the model of care is to help patients make their own decisions, with the doctor acting as a trusted adviser. So when your doctor says, "How are you doing?" you're really supposed to tell them everything you are thinking and feeling, no matter how large or small.

There are four important conversations to have with your team physician:

Conversation 1: Share Your Athletic Goals

Whether your goal is to lose twenty pounds, run a marathon, join a competitive team, or complete an Antarctic trek, the team physician's role is to assess the risks and to work with the rest of the entourage to help you achieve that goal. However, some goals are not clearly aligned with your current health. By working with a team physician you will be able to meet your goals while considering your health status. For example, if you want to enter a bike race but you have chronic back pain, a team physician might prescribe medication and physical therapy (PT), or set you up with a personal trainer who is sensitive to back issues, so that you don't aggravate your condition during the race.

There will be other times when goals may have to be postponed or reconsidered because of extreme circumstances. In those instances, the team physician's role is to provide an informed consent, even if they do not agree with your decision. For example, my patient Lori is a runner who came to see me with a stress fracture in her foot. I didn't think she should run for the next four weeks while she was in physical therapy. Lori was crushed: her goal was to run in the New York City Marathon which was only a week away.

I explained to Lori that if she ran, one of three things was likely to happen. Without a doubt she would be in constant pain throughout the race. Second, she was likely to make the condition worse by changing a stress fracture into a complete fracture, and then she would have to drop out during the race because she could not run on a broken foot. In the unlikely worst case scenario, she might hurt herself so severely that she would never be able to run again. Lori responded, "I hear you, but I've raised $10,000 for this race. I've been training for a full year to reach this goal, and it took me three years just to get the number so I could participate. What am I supposed to do?"

I totally understood where she was coming from. I knew she was disappointed and frustrated. I started to negotiate with her and tried to create perspective. I asked Lori, "Tell me more about what this race means to you. Are you willing to know that this is the last race you may ever run, or are you willing to heal and then sign up for the next marathon in Miami in January, when you would be pain free, have fun, and know that you'll be better for next year in New York?"

Luckily, Lori took my advice. But I've worked with other elite athletes who have completely ignored what I said in an effort to pursue their goals. In those instances, I often bring in another member of the entourage. I might say, "Why don't you talk to your physical therapist? Or maybe I'll talk to him. Let me get some more information." Ultimately, my goal is to help every patient see the facts so that they can make their own informed choice.

Conversation #2: Injury/Illness Prevention

During a physical, I often get asked, "Doc, what can I do to prevent injury and identify potential pitfalls in my training so I can preemptively take care of small problems before they become big issues?" This is a great conversation to have with your team physician.

For example, if you tell your team physician that you want to play soccer, she will keep an eye on your ankles and knees. If on examination they feel loose or weak, she can recommend physical therapy exercises that will build up these joints and prevent injury. Another good rule of thumb is to increase your level of game by 10 percent per week—this is for preventing injury and is also a good rule of thumb for after rehab. It can be any variable in your routine: duration, intensity, level of difficulty, surface, or competition. It also allows the body to adapt to the conditions of the sport in order to prevent overuse and injury.

Conversation #3: The Role of Supplements

I once had a patient who was told by his coach to take fourteen different nutritional supplements, because that's what all the big track stars were doing. I looked at his list as he asked, "Is this regimen going to be good for me?" I asked if I could research the list and get back to him. After I looked into the supplements more closely, I realized that many were placeboes: they weren't going to enhance his performance in any way. Some of them actually had inherent risk for kidney issues or liver issues. I was able to tell the patient exactly what could happen to his health from taking these particular supplements. I suggested that if he chose to use them, to make sure to let me know so that I could monitor his kidney and liver function.

It is imperative to disclose all supplements you take and discuss them with your doctor. Today people take supplements, including vitamins and minerals, for many reasons. It's a fact that consumers spend as many dollars on alternative medicine therapies and supplements as they do on more traditional medicine treatments. But what you might not realize is that all supplements have a medicinal value. Understanding the pro's and con's for taking them, especially if you are taking other medications, is vitally important, especially if you are having physical symptoms that cannot be explained.

Elite athletes are actually discouraged from taking supplements because of the potential for contamination with performance enhancing substances that may show up in drug testing. We also know that in 2015 the New York State Attorney General's office accused national retailer GNC and three other major supplement chains of selling herbal supplements that were fraudulent or contaminated with unlisted ingredients that could pose health risks to consumers. So if you choose to take supplements, make sure that you trust your source. One way to ensure your supplement is safe is to look for USP certified supplements (www.usp. org), which are products certified by the US Pharmacopeial Convention. The US Anti-Doping Agency has an initiative called "Supplement 411" that will give you their perspective on supplements and the ones that have potential harm. See www.usada.org/substances/supplement-411/.

Conversation #4: Your Concussion History

Concussions are a form of traumatic brain injury resulting in a disturbance in brain function caused by a direct or indirect force to the head. We used to think that in order to have a concussion it was necessary to lose consciousness. Today we know this isn't the case.

It's very easy to injure the brain because it has a very soft, fragile, almost Jell-O-like consistency encased in a very hard shell. Sadly, it is reported that there are more than 300,000 sports-related concussions sustained by athletes every year. What's worse is that there are many more that go unreported because they don't know they have experienced one.

It's also very easy to dismiss brain injury, because it's hard to see damage. But there are certain signs to look for.

There are four main categories of symptoms following concussion:

Thinking and Remembering:

- Appears dazed or stunned
- Can't recall events after the hit, bump, or fall
- Can't recall events prior to the hit, bump, or fall
- Confusion
- Difficulty learning new concepts or ideas

- Difficulty completing homework
- Difficulty making decisions
- Difficulty organizing thoughts, words, materials
- Difficulty planning, starting, doing, and finishing a task
- Decreased attention or concentration
- Difficulty remembering to do things on time
- Daydreaming more than usual
- Forgetful
- Misunderstands
- Mixes up time and/or place
- Reacts and responds slowly
- Repeats words or phrases
- Thinks slowly

Physical

- Dizzy or light-headed
- Sensitive to light or noise
- Does not "feel right"
- Develops a headache or "pressure" in the head
- Blurry or double vision
- Numbness or tingling
- Ringing in the ears
- Feels worn out or exhausted, tires easily
- Loses balance, drops things, trips
- Loses consciousness (even briefly)
- Vomits or has nausea

Emotional

- Becomes easily upset and/or loses temper
- Experiences mood swings
- Feels anxious or nervous
- Feels more stressed than usual

- Feels restless or irritable
- Feels sad or depressed
- Acts impulsively
- Increased emotional response
- Unable to cope with stress

Sleep

- Experiences restless sleep
- Feels drowsy during the day
- Has trouble falling asleep
- Sleeps less than usual
- Sleeps more than usual

Because of the plethora of symptoms, it is critical to discuss your concussion history with your doctor, and report any new symptoms as they appear. If you've had a concussion, you're more susceptible to get another on an even less impactful event. Even if you think your teammate has received a concussion, you must report it. In fact, the NFL has established a new rule where there is a dedicated third person called the head-injury spotter who sits in the stadium's upstairs viewing booth and is in direct communication with the doctors and the trainers on the field. This person is specifically watching for any change in the play style of the athletes after they take a hit.

It is highly recommended that athletes wait to return to their sport until they're fully recovered and cleared by a team physician by using the Gradual Return to Play Protocol originally created for the International Conference on Concussion in Sport in 2001. This includes the following steps. If you cannot pass these stages, you have not had full resolution of your concussion.

Stage 1: No activity—Complete physical and cognitive rest.
Stage 2: Light aerobic exercise—Walking, swimming or stationary cycling keeping exercise intensity. Less than 70 percent maximum heart rate. No resistance training.

Stage 3: Sport-specific exercise but no head impact activities.

Stage 4: Non-contact training drills, adding resistance training.

Stage 5: Full-contact practice following medical clearance.

Stage 6: Return to play.

Concussion Risk Classification

I have yet to find a sport that is not a concussion risk. The following chart lists the same sports that are included in the Sports Grid. Contact/collision sports have the highest risk, limited contact moderate risk, and noncontact low risk (but not no risk). If your activity is not listed on this chart, discuss your concussion risk with your team physician.

Contact/Collision	Limited Contact	Noncontact
Basketball	Baseball	Archery
Boxing	In-line Skating	Badminton
Cheerleading		
Diving		Bodybuilding
Field Hockey	Canoeing/Kayaking (White Water)	Bowling
Football	Fencing	Canoeing/Kayaking (Flat Water)
Ice Hockey	Field Sports (High Jump, Pole Vault)	Crew/Rowing
Lacrosse	T-Ball	Curling
Judo	Gymnastics	Ballroom Dancing
	Handball	Field Sports (Discus, Javelin, Shot Put)
Rugby	Equestrian	Golf
Ski Jumping	Racquetball	CrossFit
Soccer	Figure Skating	Weightlifting
Team Handball	Downhill Skiing	Race Walking
Water Polo	Softball	Riflery
Wrestling	Squash	Orienteering
Bobsledding	Ultimate Frisbee	Running

Contact/Collision	Limited Contact	Noncontact
Luge	Volleyball	Sailing
Karate	Windsurfing/surfing	Scuba Diving
Krav Maga	Climbing	Hiking
Dodgeball	Water Skiing	Swimming
Street/Roller Hockey	Cross-country Skiing	Table Tennis
Parkour	Dance Team	Tennis
Ultimate Frisbee	Mountain Biking	Field Events (Jumping)
Auto racing	Triathlon	Weight lifting
Motocross	Speed Cycling	Arm-wrestling
BMX Cycling	Skateboarding	Stair Climbing
	Snowboarding	Kayaking
	Speed Skating	Rowing
	Road Cycling	Paddle-boarding
	Cricket	Archery
	BASE Jumping	Fly Fishing
	Hang Gliding	Synchronized Swimming
	Paintball	Bocce Ball
	Obstacle Racing	Bowling
		Darts
		Shuffleboard
		Skeet Shooting

Meet Paralympic Medalist Tucker Dupree

Tucker Dupree is a blind swimmer and one of the most inspiring athletes I've met under difficult circumstances. In the London 2012 Paralympics he won three medals: a silver and two bronze. But the year before, when I was working at the US Olympic Training Center, I had to treat Tucker on my very first day. He was swimming in a lane with another swimmer and they collided. Both athletes received severe concussions. As I followed their progress over the course of the next two weeks, Tucker had taken my advice to heart, much more so than the other athlete. He made sure not to use technology during his recovery, including listening to music. He made sure to get plenty of rest. By the time I left, Tucker was back in the pool and training; the other swimmer wasn't doing as well, and was still on the sidelines.

Tucker has a rare disease called Leber's Hereditary Optic Neuropathy, or LHON, a genetic mutation that started affecting his eyesight when he was seventeen. Eventually, it caused 80 percent vision loss. Today Tucker is twenty-five years old, living in Chicago, and training for his third Paralympics: the 2016 games in Rio de Janeiro, Brazil. Since I met him he has broken a world record in the 100 Backstroke and hopes to win the 100 Backstroke and the 50 Freestyle.

When I interviewed him in 2015 about the relationship he has with his team physician, Tucker told me, "In order to stay on top, one of my primary relationships in life is with my doctors. The fact is my body is the vehicle that I use to compete in a sport, so being honest with someone that hopefully has your best interest in mind is a partnership you can't jeopardize. Creating an honest partnership so that I'm using my doctor as a sounding board is only going to help my progression."

During our interview I reminded him about the day we met, and I asked how his relationship with me helped him recover from his concussion. Tucker told me, "The fact that I was only going to be at the USOTC for a short training session, I knew I had to maximize my time in order for me to be successful. I didn't need to fight the giant in the room by pretending that I was healthy. I didn't think it would be in my best interest to fight all that was going on. I chose to listen to you, comply, and we figured out how I could progress. I knew we weren't reinventing the wheel. I didn't have some crazy rare condition. I had a concussion. The biggest decision I had to make was saying, 'Okay, what do I need to do? How do we move forward?' and then following what you had to say. That was pretty much key."

I then asked him what he considered to be the most important elements of the doctor/patient relationship. Tucker told me, "Trust your doc. You want the doctor to have your best interest. That's part of the reason you go there. The fact that they went to school more than most people is probably the best reason to be honest. Doctors know all about the human body and have that edge on you. If they are able to work with you and you're honest, and that channel is open you are going to be a lot more successful.

"The point of being a Paralympian is overcoming obstacles but also having no fear. We don't let our disabilities define who we are. Saying 'Okay, I'm open to anything that's going to make me successful' is what makes you an elite athlete, but also a Paralympic athlete. So I don't think I have a different relationship with my doctors than any other athlete. At the end of the day I'm still a human. The fact is, the doctor is there to help with your needs regardless of your health. I consider my condition a very minute disability compared to some other athletes.

"You can be as big as you want. Live your life like a champion. Being extraordinary is something that is basically the point of my athletic career. I've had people tell me, 'Your disability won't hold you back and you'll never be ordinary.' Every time I race and every time I'm able to be successful is showing them that they're right and I was able to be extraordinary."

The Team Physician Is the Quarterback for Your Health

A team physician will monitor your health at all times. If you are currently healthy and ready to play, the team physician is a role that stays in the background, and is ready and available for you. Knowing your physician is there for you should provide you a level of comfort and therefore less insecurity. Interestingly, I got fewer calls from my patients when I practiced concierge medicine than when I was operating in a more traditional office setting. When my patients had my cell phone number and immediate access to me they were less likely to panic and contact me, unless they were having a true emergency.

A good team physician also knows that they can't do everything alone. They'll make sure that you are covering the roles of the dietitian, the athletic trainer, the physical therapist, etc., and then orchestrate your program to make sure all of these roles work in concert. After each referred role provides their expertise, the team physician communicates with them to ensure the right care was properly delivered. For example, if an athlete requires a dietitian to change his or her eating habits and either gain or lose weight, the team physician will make sure that this advice fits with the overall wellness plan and does not conflict with other treatments.

In Case of Injury

Injury or illness is inevitable to being human, and something elite athletes deal with all the time. As soon as they recognize that poor health is hampering their performance, or putting them at risk, they see their team physician. The following explains how to evaluate an injury so that you can make an informed decision as to whether you need to go to the doctor, go to the emergency room, or just treat yourself.

Go to the ER or Call 911: Recognizing Life-Threatening Injury or Pain

- Any injury that threatens the loss of a limb
- Back pain where you cannot get out of bed or that is getting worse with rest
- Bleeding that cannot be controlled after applying five minutes of constant pressure
- Broken bones—any bone deformity with swelling and bruising after trauma
- Chest pain and/or shortness of breath
- Head trauma with loss of consciousness
- Head trauma with headache that is worsening
- Head trauma accompanied by numbness, tingling, or weakness
- Neck pain with loss of range of motion after trauma
- Passing out

Call the Doctor: Recognizing Illness or Injury that Is Urgent but Not Life-Threatening

- Fever greater than 101.4°F that does not respond to over-the-counter fever reducers—aspirin, acetaminophen (Tylenol), or NSAIDs like ibuprofen (Motrin, Advil)
- Injury or illness that is not resolving with rest after three days
- Pain that is not responding to rest and over-the-counter pain medications: acetaminophen, ibuprofen, naproxen, aspirin
- Sustain head injury but are awake and alert, with no numbness, tingling, weakness, headache, or blurry vision
- Swelling and loss of range in motion of a joint after injury that is not responding to rest, ice, compression, or elevation after twenty-four hours

Time-Out: Ice versus Heat for Treating Pain

There are no studies to support the use of either one, although I use ice and heat for different applications. My rule of thumb is for the first twenty-four to forty-eight hours after an acute injury, use ice for twenty minutes on the hour along with some elevation and compression. This is part of the RICE method: Rest, Ice, Compression, Elevation. Compression means to put on, for example, an Ace bandage. The ice is thought to reduce inflammation that overly ensues and reduce pain.

I use heat for more chronic muscular tension or muscle spasm. Moist heat will actually help muscles relax. If you have a chronically tense upper back, getting in the shower and using hot water with the beating action, like a massage, can be very effective.

Wait and See

- Back or limb pain secondary to injury without a loss of range or motion
- Fever greater than 101.4°F that responds to over-the-counter fever reducers
- Pain that responds to over-the-counter pain relievers

Developing a Recovery Protocol

Once the initial crisis is over, athletes work with their team physician to develop a recovery plan. I strongly recommend that you do not play or train when you are hurt or significantly sick. Let your coach (if you have one) know that you will be out for whatever time the doctor recommends. Then, stick with the plan.

As I mentioned earlier, having an injury does not always mean being completely inactive. A good team physician will prescribe rehabilitation as soon as possible to ensure a quick return to full activity. He or she may also recommend cross training on other body parts while you heal, or engage in a modified activity. For example, if you have a simple ankle sprain you may be able to cross train with cycling or swimming while you recover as long as you do not put pressure on the outside of the ankle by making side to side motions. Straight line and non-weight bearing movements are allowed as tolerated to pain. I ask patients to pedal with their heel on the affected ankle instead of the ball of the foot, or swim with a buoy placed between their legs. Concussion is the one exception: you will need to shut down your training completely until you are symptom-free.

The team physician also determines the "return to play" guidelines. Having grown up the son of a physician, I saw many 'home remedies' that my father used, including limiting my activity whenever I got hurt. His advice was typically, "If it hurts to do it, don't do it." Today, a team physician will know how to keep you active as you recover from injury. Often, staying immobilized can prolong the healing process. For example, for some simple broken bones the textbook answer was to keep it in a cast for four to six weeks. These days I often put on a removable brace for ten days to two weeks, and then reassess the fracture's stability. Then I slowly allow the physical therapist to wean the patient off the brace while starting physical therapy. This allows for early mobilization that will not disrupt the bone healing. This minimizes muscle stiffness and weakness that would definitely occur if the limb was casted for the entire time.

Injury and rehabilitation are part of being an athlete, so learning how to accept it and deal with it is an important skill. Eventually, you or your teammates will see how well you dealt with it, and they will view you as a leader and source of strength.

Home Remedies: Treatments You Can Do on Your Own

While you can't really be a team physician, you can learn to think like one. There are many instances when you can treat yourself. For example, if you have a muscle strain from training, if it's not impairing your function, you can try over-the-counter remedies discussed above. You can also try the RICE method outlined above. Protect any injured body parts until they are completely healed. But if the pain doesn't go away in a couple of days, go ahead and see your doctor.

However, athletes have to be careful with some over-the-counter treatments. A lot of them can interfere with your athletic performance:

- NSAIDs (like ibuprofen or naproxen) are not recommended for long distance runners (greater than four hours) because it can affect kidney function and lead to *hyponatremia* (low sodium in blood). Its use can also lead to GI bleeding in anyone if taken too often. It is also thought to lead to kidney failure if taken in too high a dose or taken chronically.
- Cold medications containing pseudoephedrine can cause anyone to have high heart rates and increases in blood pressure. It can lead to hand tremors and feeling jittery. This is because it has a stimulant effect. Pseudoephedrine has a conditional status on

the banned substance list according to the World Anti-Doping Agency (WADA), and elite athletes rarely take it, and never take it during competition.

- Diphenhydramine (Benadryl) can make most people feel drowsy and some jittery and wired.

Typical Ailments	Recommended Course of Action
Allergic rash	• Aveeno bath for itching • Hydrocortisone cream or Benadryl cream
Back ache	• Ice 20 minutes every waking hour for 24 to 48 hours. • Moist heat (bath or hot water bottle) for 1 hour if chronic or you experience muscle spasm. • 3 to 4 times per day use heat patches if needed, like ThermaCare. • Topical cream like Icy Hot can be helpful.
Common cold or allergies	• Sinus massage (light massage above, on side, and below eyes and on nose) for one minute 5 to 6 times per day. • Saline nasal spray. • Over-the-counter remedies like Mucinex to thin secretions. • Antihistamines for allergies; steam treatment (hot shower).
Diarrhea	• Stay hydrated with a mixture of 1/2 electrolyte replacement drink, 1/2 water. • Refrain from using Imodium—let body get rid of the bug.
Headache	• Lightly massage neck and scalp. • Over-the-counter pain relievers
Joint aches	• Arnica cream or ointment • Glucosamine/chondroitin • Over-the-counter pain reliever (try acetaminophen before NSAIDs)
Muscle strain	• Arnica cream or ointment • Over-the-counter pain reliever (try acetaminophen before NSAID)
Nausea	• Ginger/ginger ale

Be Your Own Medical Researcher

Team physicians are constantly researching the latest trends and treatments. If you want to think like a doctor, you'll need to be able to research medical information and understand how to process it in order to make educated decisions about your health.

With all the medical information available on the Internet, the question of how we separate what's useful from what's not has become increasingly important. Some of it is thoughtfully produced and accurate, and some of it is just plain wrong. If you'd like to research a medical concern, the American Academy of Family Physicians patient website (familydoctor.org) has basic information about every condition you may have. HealthTap can also answer very specific questions that patients pose: doctors post their answers without really giving medical advice. Another great resource is the American College of Sports Medicine's website: www.acsm.org/access-public-information/search-by-topic.

For a second, deeper reading you can try PubMed, which is the National Institutes of Health website that lists all of the recently published medical studies in abstract form. That means you can get an overview of the latest medical information—but it can be a bit overwhelming and difficult to read if you don't have experience with medical studies. If you want to pay for the same exact material that a doctor would be looking at, try UptoDate.com. It is a subscription service that provides helpful, thorough summaries of many conditions. The Medical Library Association considers the following to be the most useful consumer health websites: Centers for Disease Control and Prevention, Healthfinder, Kidshealth, MayoClinic, and MedlinePlus.

Some people like to view chat threads about certain conditions, and while they can give some information it is difficult to differentiate if the information is correct. I find chat sites can lead readers down the path of unnecessary fear, especially for athletes who research supplements—there is a lot of false information out there.

Use your research to generate thoughtful questions for your team physician. Do not use the web as a means to diagnose any condition. While it's nice to know the treatment options, don't become biased as to what is best for you until you know what your doctor thinks.

CHAPTER 3
THE PHYSICAL THERAPIST

No matter what the injury—unless it's completely debilitating—I'm going to be the same player I've always been. I'll figure it out. I'll make some tweaks, some changes, but I'm still coming.

—Kobe Bryant

Cameron was twenty-eight years old when he sullenly limped into my office. He had signed up for an IRONMAN triathlon and he desperately wanted to participate, but during his training he had developed a sharp pain on the outside of his left knee whenever he ran. He had already tried Pilates and yoga in an attempt to stretch out his leg, and although he was working with a running coach, he was not getting better.

I immediately noticed that he had iliotibial band (IT) syndrome of the knee, and his weak hips were causing his problem. I recommended that he follow the same physical therapy (PT) protocol that I give my elite athletes. Cameron needed to strengthen his hip muscles which would then change his gait and reduce his pain.

We didn't have a lot of time; the race was just five weeks away. Cameron worked really hard with the physical therapist in my office, coming in two or three times a week. The therapist taught him how to strengthen his hip muscles with resistance band exercises, stretching with a stability ball, and rolling his IT band with a foam roller. He also learned how to properly tape up his knee before he ran in order to change its biomechanics and take some pressure off the joint. At the end of four weeks Cameron was up to running nineteen miles at a stretch pain-free.

Physical therapists diagnose injuries and then use an array of techniques, tools, and modalities to rehabilitate or fix muscular and balance issues so that you can quickly return to playing. Elite athletes know that the riskier the activity, the more likely they're going to need PT. That's why they frequently have a physical therapist as part of their entourage. But what they often don't share is that these same athletes also know that they can also improve their performance by working with a physical therapist to create a proactive program for injury prevention. This not only keeps athletes healthy, it improves their flexibility and strengthens muscles, which can reduce the risk of injury. This type of program prepares the body well to support the stresses of each particular sport. For example, the explosive movements of basketball, which require rapidly generating high forces require a stronger upper core, as compared to the movements required for bowling.

Professional physical therapists are a huge asset to your entourage, and it is a role that can easily be filled. Your team physician can recommend a good one, especially if you are currently suffering from an acute injury. However, it is also a role that you can take on for yourself. In this chapter you will learn how to identify common anatomical weaknesses that can predispose you to injury, learn how to perform rehabilitation (rehab) exercises for the most common injuries, and most important, learn how to "pre-habilitate" (prehab): how to strengthen the specific muscles your athletic endeavors require, whether you are recovering from injury or just want to prevent one from happening.

My unique prehab routine includes three critical components: strength, flexibility, and balance training. Strength training establishes your physical foundation so you can generate adequate force. Flexibility training ensures that you are pliable enough to have optimal range of motion. Stability is important for maintaining balance even when moving quickly. Once you've mastered these exercises, you will be able to build on your success with a more advanced strength training workout in the next chapter.

When to Use Physical Therapy

If you are currently injured and applying ice, heat, or stretching doesn't relieve your pain, or if it doesn't get better in a day or two with relative rest, then it's time to see your team physician so that you can diagnose what's going on. Then, you can start to take your recovery into your own hands by either seeing a physical therapist or discussing the exercises recommended in this chapter with your doctor.

Once you have a proper diagnosis, take it slowly and gently as you try the following suggestions. You can expect a certain amount of relieving pain, such as the way you'll feel when you are getting a massage and a muscle knot in the neck is released. However, if the massage is too aggressive and the pain too intense, it can put the muscle into spasm. Therefore, it is important to be able to recognize the fine line between relieving pain and true pain. "True" pain is typically sharp in nature, limits muscle/joint flexibility, and/or causes a radiating pain. "Relieving" pain is often described as a soreness that increasingly feels better during the treatment; it increases muscle/joint flexibility, and does not cause radiating or lasting pain. Remember, experiencing true pain is not a part of recovery.

Physical Therapy Tools

Physical therapists use a variety of tools that are easy to find and use for both rehab and prehab. Use them carefully: these tools can end up hurting you if you use them too aggressively. You can find most of these tools at a sports equipment store, or on the Internet.

Foam Roller: A foam roller is a stretching tool that is used when you have a restriction in motion. It is roughly six inches wide and one or two feet long or longer. Foam rollers are used by gently rolling the constricted muscle over the roller, which then allows the fascia—the thin piece of connective tissue that covers the muscles to gently stretch. For example, if you suffer from occasional low back pain, you can roll over the lower back to get a deeper stretch. Originally they were made out of foam, but today you can find similar products made of hard plastic.

Stability Ball: The stability ball is commonly known by its brand name, Swiss Ball, and is used to strengthen the core muscles or when you need to improve your balance. It's about two feet round and bouncy when you sit on it. Athletes use the stability ball to practice balance or stretch out over it. It creates an unstable platform and it works your body by challenging it to create stability, core strength, and balance. For example, you could lie on a stability ball and try to stay on top of it as a means to engage your core muscles.

Trigger Point Massager: Back Buddy and Thera Cane are two brands of trigger point massager. It is a long staff that is covered with knobs that can be used to massage *trigger points*, such as the knots that form in your neck or shoulders when you have been working at a desk for a long period of time. These knots form because they have been deprived of proper movement and now have decreased blood supply and lymph flow. The small knobs relieve the trigger point or knot by applying pressure. To use it, hold it in one hand and position it according to the trigger point map provided, applying pressure to those areas.

Resistance Bands: Resistance bands, like the TheraBand or REP Band brands, are lightweight latex (there is also latex-free version for those who are sensitive or allergic) exercise bands that come in color-coded levels that signify different tensiles, or strengths of increasing tension. Most muscles can be exercised with resistance bands. Make sure you start with a band that allows you to feel challenged. My general rule there is that you should be able to do fifteen repetitions, and do it two sets without causing a pain. When this gets too easy, it's time to switch to the next level up of resistance band.

Lacrosse Ball: The standard lacrosse ball can be used to stretch muscles and release deep, nagging, knotty areas that you need to try to roll out when stretching or even a foam roller isn't effective. It can also get into tight areas where the foam roller may be too big to properly target. For example, athletes commonly use a lacrosse ball to release the front outer portion of the hip, known as the *tensor fascia lata muscle*, which can get tight with repetitive hip rotation. You can also use a standard softball or even a tennis ball if the lacrosse ball causes an increase in pain.

Stretching Belt: A stretching belt can be used to stretch out individual muscles. Unlike a resistance band, a stretching belt does not actually stretch: it's more like a strap or a rope. To use it you typically attach it to a limb of the body and then pull to create a maximal, controllable stretch. Stretching belts come in various lengths; I always recommend getting the longest one possible because they come with loops or a buckle that can be set to a short length if needed.

Balance Board or Stability Trainer: A stability trainer is used to create instability when you stand on it so that you can improve balance, equilibrium, and *proprioception*; proprioception is the unconscious perception of movement and spatial orientation. It is typically a foam pad that has a ribbed, anti-slip surface. They come in different levels of firmness: start with the easiest one (firm is easier, softer is more difficult) then progress from there. Another option is the BOSU Balance Trainer.

Anatomical Weaknesses That Cause Injury

Over the years I have seen almost every possible injury described in my sport medicine textbooks. Surprisingly, the vast majority are injuries that could have been completely preventable, such as overuse injuries. Overuse injuries can be attributed to key anatomical weaknesses. No matter what overuse injury my athletes have incurred, they are typically accompanied by one or more key muscle imbalances that contributed to the problem. In other words, the injury was waiting to happen.

We all need to learn how to "pre-habilitate," to keep specific muscles strong in the long term. Most physical therapists will recommend that in order to participate in any sport you need to get strong first. You can accomplish this by strengthening the key muscles that are related to the most common anatomical weaknesses. It's important to make the connection between your sport and the various muscles upon which it relies. At the same time, it's worth any athlete's time to make sure that these muscles listed below are all as strong as possible.

Paraspinal Neck Muscles: The muscles that cross the upper back and the back of the neck. These muscles typically become fatigued from sitting in front of a computer. Sports that require a strong upper core—the chest through the shoulders, upper back and neck—require strengthening this area.

Rotator Cuff: The set of muscles that connect your arm to your shoulder blade. These muscles weaken with poor posture and rounded shoulders (hunched forward). Athletes who play sports like tennis and baseball that require arm movements at shoulder height or higher frequently injure this muscle group. Additionally, sports that require a strong upper core—the chest through the shoulders, upper back and neck—require strengthening this area.

Serratus Anterior: The muscle that connects each shoulder blade to the side of the chest wall. This muscle becomes weak due to a shoulder muscle imbalance. Again, athletes who play sports like tennis and baseball that require arm movements at shoulder height or higher frequently injure this muscle group. Additionally, sports that require a strong upper core—the chest through the shoulders, upper back and neck—require strengthening this area.

Lower Trapezius and Rhomboid Muscles: The muscles between the shoulder blades in the mid back. These become weak due to computer use and poor posture, with shoulders hunched forward. They need to be strengthened to support all sports that involve the upper core. Of all the anatomical weaknesses, these muscles are the most important to strengthen because they keep the shoulder blades in balance so that the shoulders do not become rounded or project forward.

Back Extensor Muscle Group: The set of deep muscles that lie close to the spinal column. These muscles keep us upright and balanced. They are important to strengthen to ensure upper and lower core balance.

Hip Abductors (Gluteus Medius): Lower core muscles that surround the outer part of the hip socket. They can become weakened from inactivity or prolonged sitting. It is important to strengthen them for lower core stability and leg alignment, especially for running sports like soccer, lacrosse, and running in general.

Maintaining Balance and Coordinating Movement

Balance exercises improve *proprioception*, the ability to coordinate movement without volitionally thinking about it. For example, Roger Federer's incredible footwork shows how proprioception truly works. He has the best footwork in tennis because his sense of balance, movement, and equilibrium is so fine-tuned—it's as if he glides across the court. His coordination is phenomenal, and he has the knack to be in the right position at the right time. His proprioception I believe is one of the biggest keys to his seemingly effortless effort in setting up for his tennis shots.

Without excellent proprioception athletes have to think about every single movement and step, creating an inefficiency that decreases reaction time, lessens the forces generated by their bodies, and increases their chances of injury. As we age, we naturally lose our sense of proprioception, and if we don't maintain this ability we are at increased risk for falls. Studies show that proprioception is maintained and gained by doing activities that work on the brain's control of postural muscles. These exercises develop fine and gross motor skills in coordinating movement. The proprioception exercises below will help develop this vital part of your athletic self for those sports where it is most necessary.

The Importance of Stretching

Stretching is critical for proper muscle function because it brings a muscle to its full optimal length. It is used to ensure proper range of motion for joints, maintain the best elasticity of the muscle and fascia, and to decrease pain. Muscles need to be adequately flexible in order to contract with a maximal force. If the muscle is not properly stretched it will not function optimally; you will not have maximal strength; and you are more likely to injure it.

One trick physical therapists teach is to add Proprioceptive Neuromuscular Facilitation, or Muscle Energy as DOs call it, to stretches in order to make them more effective. Every muscle in your body contracts to create a force. This technique allows the muscles to achieve their optimal length in a superior fashion compared to passive stretching.

For each stretch, bring the muscle into a full stretch but not to the point of pain. Then activate, or *contract* the muscle without moving your position for five seconds. This is known as an *isometric contraction*. Use a low level of force to activate the muscle, which is defined as using less than 25 percent of your maximal force of contraction. You should feel the contraction but your muscle should not tremble. Then relax the muscle for three seconds. Repeat this process three times. Afterward, stretch the muscle again, but this time without contraction, to its maximal point of stretch and hold for ten seconds. This is called a *passive stretch*.

At no point during this exercise should you experience pain: if you feel pain it means that you are either stretching too far or contracting too hard. When you are done you will have an increased range of motion, more than if you had done plain stretching.

The Injury Prevention Workout Grid

Use the following variation of the Sports Grid to determine which specific muscles you must strengthen, based on your sport. These exercises will help prevent injury and will give you a solid foundation on which you will build additional muscular strength that we will work on in Chapter 4.

Let's take running for example. Some of the muscles a runner will need to work on are intuitive, but others are counterintuitive. For example, runners like Cameron often suffer from IT band syndrome, which is a pain on the outside of the knee that is not caused by a structural abnormality or injury. Therefore, on the grid you'll see that runners need to focus on exercise groups 2, 3, and 4: these are the exercises for the back, the lower core, and proprioception respectively. By strengthening the lower core and back and enhancing flexibility and proprioception, runners can help protect the lower kinetic chain that includes the hip, thigh, knee, calf, ankle, and foot. The muscles, ligaments, fascia, and tendons surrounding the knee will optimally function by having muscles that are strong, flexible, and in balance with the entire lower kinetic chain.

These prehab exercises are identified as follows:

Group 1: Upper Core
Group 2: Back
Group 3: Lower Core
Group 4: Proprioception

First, find your sport on the grid. Remember your sector number; it will become more important as you progress in the book. Then, complete the prehab exercise routine two to three times a week in addition to your workout. If you're thinking about switching sports, become proficient in these exercises before taking on the new sport, and certainly before ramping up to the strengthening exercises featured in Chapter 4. You will know that you are proficient in these exercises when you can do them all with consistency and with minimal effort over a two-week period.

Sector 1	Sector 2	Sector 3
• Arm-wrestling 1,2 • Bobsledding 1,2,3 • Cheerleading 1,2,3,4 • Climbing 1,2,3,4 • Dance Team 1,2,3,4 • Field Events (throwing) 1,2,3,4 • Gymnastics 1,2,3,4 • Judo 1,2,3,4 • Karate 1,2,3,4 • Krav Maga 1,2,3,4 • Luge 1,2,3 • Sailing 1,2,3,4 • Water Skiing 1,2,3,4 • Weight Lifting 1,2,3,4 • Windsurfing 1,2,3,4	• Ballroom Dance 2,3,4 • Body-building 1,2,3 • Cycling—BMX 1,2,3,4 • Downhill Skiing 2,3,4 • Mountain Biking 1,2,3,4 • Skateboarding 2,3,4 • Snowboarding 2,3,4 • Wrestling 1,2,3,4	• Boxing 1,2,3,4 • Canoeing 1,2 • CrossFit 1,2,3,4 • Kayaking 1,2 • Rowing 1,2,3 • Speed (Track) Cycling 2,3,4 • Speed Skating 2,3,4 • Stair Climbing 2,3 • Triathlon 1,2,3,4 • Water Polo 1,2,3,4
Sector 4	Sector 5	Sector 6
• Archery 1,2, 4 • Auto Racing 1,2 • BASE Jumping 2,3 • Diving 1,2,3,4 • Equestrian 1,2,3 • Fly fishing 1,2 • Hang Gliding 1,2 • Motocross 1,2,3,4	• Dodgeball 1,2,3,4 • Figure Skating 2,3,4 • Football 1,2,3,4 • Field Events (jumping) 2,3,4 • Obstacle Racing 1,2,3,4 • Parkour 1,2,3,4 • Paintball 1,2,3,4 • Rugby 1,2,3,4 • Running (speed-sprint) 2,3,4 • Surfing 1,2,3,4 • Synchronized Swimming 1,2,3,4	• Basketball 1,2,3,4 • Cross-country Skiing (skating technique) 1,2,3,4 • Road Cycling 2,3,4 • Ice Hockey 1,2,3,4 • Lacrosse 1,2,3,4 • Paddle Boarding 1,2,3,4 • Running (5K to 10K) 2,3,4 • Street/Roller Hockey 1,2,3,4 • Swimming 1,2,3 • Team Handball 1,2,3,4

Sector 7	Sector 8	Sector 9
• Bocce Ball 1,2 • Bowling 1,2,3,4 • Cricket 1,2,3,4 • Darts 1,2 • Golf 1,2,3 • Riflery 1,2 • Scuba Diving 2,3 • Shuffleboard 1,2 • Skeet Shooting 1,2,4	• Baseball 1,2,3,4 • Fencing 1,2,3,4 • Hiking 2,3,4 • Softball 1,2,3,4 • Table Tennis 1,2,3,4 • T-Ball 1,2,3,4 • Volleyball 1,2,3,4	• Badminton 1,2,3,4 • Cross-country Skiing (classic technique) 1,2,3,4 • Field Hockey 1,2,3,4 • Handball 1,2,3,4 • In-line Skating 2,3,4 • Orienteering 2,3,4 • Race Walking 2,3,4 • Racquetball 1,2,3,4 • Running (long distance) 2,3,4 • Soccer 2,3,4 • Squash 1,2,3,4 • Tennis 1,2,3,4 • Ultimate Frisbee 1,2,3,4

Group 1: Upper Core Exercises

These exercises address the key areas that are most often deficient in strength and flexibility in the upper core, which includes the neck, chest, and upper back. By mastering them your head, shoulders, and arms will be properly supported at all times, reducing the likelihood of injury.

The Chin Tuck

To start: Stand straight, maintaining the best posture you can with your hands by your sides.

1. Place three fingers from one hand on your chin. Don't let your chin move up or down.
2. Gently push head/chin straight back until you cannot move your head back any further. Contract your head forward into fingers

isometrically with a low level of force for five seconds, then relax for three seconds.

3. Push head/chin back to the new point of maximal stretch, then isometrically contract head forward into fingers with a low level of force for five secs, then relax for three seconds.
4. Repeat Step 3, and then at the end do a passive stretch for ten seconds.
5. Complete two sets.

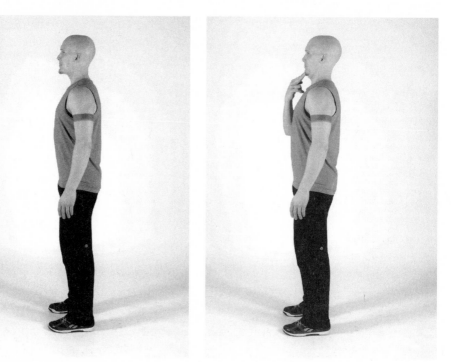

External Rotation Rotator Cuff Exercise

To start: For left shoulder, hold a resistance band in your right hand or attach it to a stationary, secured object like a stair case railing or secure door knob. In a standing position, secure the other end of the band in your left hand with your left upper arm pressed against your abdomen with your elbow bent. Position the band at a 45-degree angle in front of your abdomen.

1. Pull the band away from your abdomen to reach 45 degrees on the side of your body.
2. Hold for three seconds, and then allow it to slowly return to the starting position.

Repeat 15 times for one set; complete two sets. Switch to the right shoulder, then repeat sequence.

Note: Keep your upper arm and the angle in your elbow constant. The resistance is dependent on how far you stand from where the band is secured—make sure to stand where you are comfortable enough to do 15 repetitions without compromising form and feeling fatigued toward the end. If you are too close the exercise will be too easy. If you are too far, then the exercise may be too difficult.

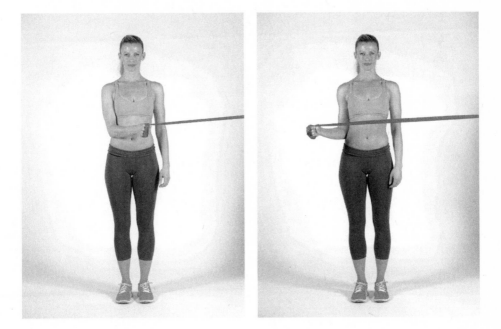

Push-Up Plus

To start: Place your hands on the floor, slightly wider than shoulder width apart. Extend legs behind with toes on the floor.

1. With your arms fully extended, bend elbows to 90 degrees or lightly touch your chest to the floor, lowering your upper body. Hold for three seconds, then go back to the start position.
2. Contract your shoulders downward toward your feet without moving them (this activates your *latissimus dorsi muscles,* the muscles in the middle and low back that attach to the upper arms. Your shoulder blades should come together.
3. Push up and straighten out your arms while rotating only your shoulder blades; bring your shoulder blades apart. This activates the *serratus anterior muscles,* the muscles that connect your shoulder blades to your chest wall.
4. Lower your body and return to the starting position.

Repeat 15 times for one set; complete two sets.

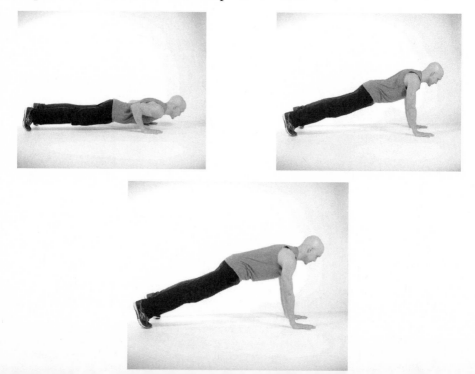

Rows with Resistance Band

To start: Stand with your arms at your sides. Secure a resistance band to a point higher than your head, like the top of a door. Grab an end in each hand. Keep shoulders relaxed and low throughout the movement. Maintain a good center of gravity by keeping knees slightly bent and feet shoulder width apart.

1. Pull down the band with both arms until your hands are by your waist with bent elbows behind you. Hold this position for three seconds.
2. Slowly return your hands to the starting position.

Repeat 15 times for one set; complete two sets.

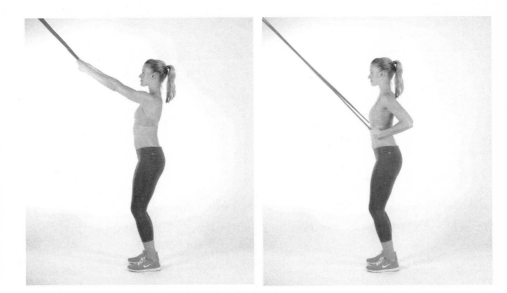

Straight Arm Pull Down with Resistance Band

To start: Stand with your arms at your sides. Secure a resistance band to a point higher than your head, like the top of a door. Grab an end in each hand. Keep shoulders relaxed and low throughout the movement.

Maintain a good center of gravity by keeping knees slightly bent and feet shoulder width apart.
1. Pull down the band with straight arms until your hands are behind you. Hold this position for three seconds.
2. Slowly return your hands to the starting position.

Repeat 15 times for one set; complete two sets.

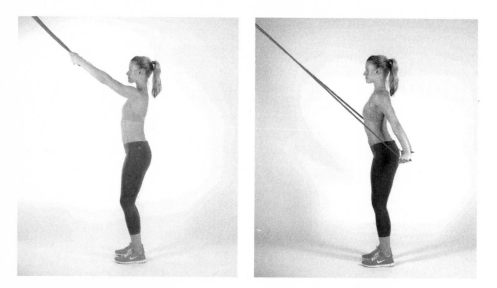

Levator Scapulae Stretch

To start: Stand with good posture and head erect.
1. Take the index and middle fingers on your right hand and reach behind the left side of your head.
2. Pull your head down toward your right side creating a 45-degree angle. At the point of maximal stretch isometrically contract head upward with a low of level force for five seconds, then relax for three seconds.
3. Pull head down again to new point of maximal stretch then isometrically contract head upward with a low level of force for five seconds, then relax for three seconds.

4. Repeat Step 3, then do a passive stretch for ten seconds.
5. Do two sets, then repeat the exercise on the opposite side.

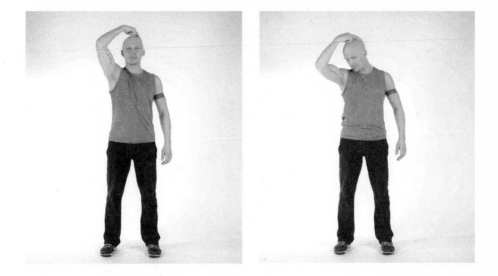

Posterior Shoulder Stretch

To start: Stand with good posture.

1. Take your right forearm and place on front of your left elbow.
2. Pull your right arm across your body by using your left arm to pull it across your body, in order to feel a stretch in the back of shoulder. Continue to maintain good posture and stand forward. At the point of maximal stretch isometrically contract your right arm away from your body with a low level of force for five seconds, and then relax for three seconds.
3. Pull your right arm again in same direction and feel new point of maximal stretch and isometrically contract your arm away with a low level of force for five seconds, then relax for three seconds.
4. Repeat Step 3, then do a passive stretch for ten seconds.
5. Do two sets, and then repeat the exercise on the opposite side.

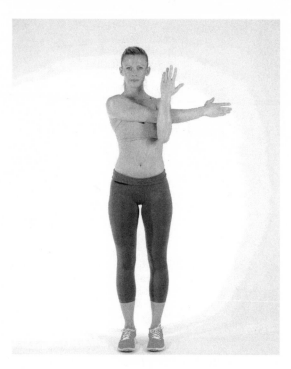

Pectoralis Stretch

To start: Position two chairs parallel to each other. Get down on your knees with the chairs on either side of you. Make sure to have enough space in between the chairs for you to fit your body between them.

1. Place your forearms on each chair seat.
2. Lean downward so your upper body is below the level of the seat of the chair to the point of maximal stretch. Isometrically contract your arms downward with a low level of force for five seconds, then relax for three seconds.
3. Lean downward in same direction and feel new point of maximal stretch. Isometrically contract your arms downward with a low level of force for five seconds, then relax for three seconds.
4. Repeat Step 3, then do passive stretch for ten seconds.
5. Do two sets.

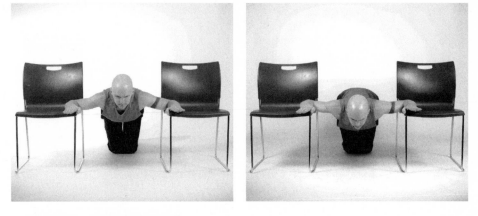

Latissimus Dorsi Stretch

To start: Kneel in front of a chair.

1. Place your hands on the sides of the seat of the chair with your arms fully extended.
2. Lean downward so you can feel the stretch in the back and sides of your upper body. Pull the chair isometrically toward you with a low level of force for five seconds, then relax for three seconds.
3. Lean downward and feel the new point of maximal stretch. Pull the chair isometrically toward you with a low level of force for five seconds, then relax for three seconds.
4. Repeat Step 3, then do a passive stretch for ten seconds.
5. Do two sets.

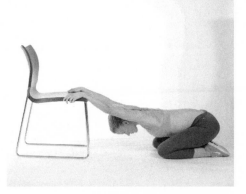

Group 2: Back Exercises

These exercises address the weaknesses in the back by strengthening the upper, mid, and low back, and increasing flexibility in the low back and pelvis.

Supermans

To start: This exercise is a series of four different movements. Lay on your stomach. Rest arms, legs, and head on the floor.
1. Lift your left arm and right leg straight into the air so that your left shoulder and right hip are off the ground three to five inches.
2. Hold for three seconds, and then lower to original starting position.

Repeat 15 times for one set; complete two sets. Switch to right arm and left leg. Repeat 15 times for one set; complete two sets.

3. Once you are comfortable with the exercise above, continue to add these movements. Lift both arms straight into the air to the point of raising both shoulders off the ground three to five inches.
4. Hold for three seconds, and then lower to original starting position. Repeat 15 times for one set; complete two sets.
5. Lift both legs straight into the air to the point of raising both hips off the ground three to five inches.
6. Hold for three seconds, and then lower to original starting position. Repeat 15 times for one set; complete two sets.

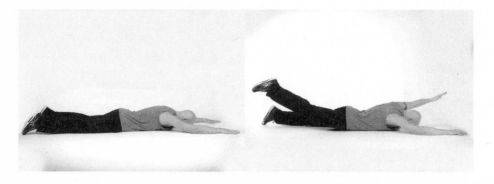

7. Lift your both arms and legs straight into the air to the point of raising both shoulders and hips off the ground three to five inches.
8. Hold for three seconds, then lower to original starting position. Repeat 15 times for one set; complete two sets.

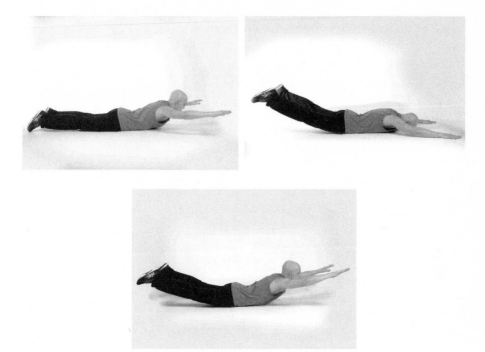

Lumbar Rotation Stretch

To start: Lie down on your back.

1. Take your right leg with a slightly bent knee and pull it over the left side of your body with your left hand.
2. Keep your right arm stretched away from your body and on the floor. Feel the stretch in your lumbar spine. Contract your right leg toward the right side of your body isometrically with a low level of force for five seconds, then relax for three seconds. You can put a weight on your foot or wedge your foot under a stationary object like a couch, or put your foot against a wall.

3. Pull the left leg farther and feel the new point of maximal stretch in your lumbar spine. Contract your right leg toward the right side of your body isometrically with a low level of force for five seconds, then relax for three seconds.
4. Repeat Step 3, then do passive stretch for ten seconds.
5. Do two sets. Switch sides and repeat.

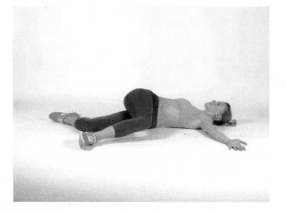

Piriformis Stretch

To start: Lie on your back.
1. Place your left lower leg on your right thigh near your knee. Bend your right hip while keeping your left leg on your right lower thigh.
2. Place both hands behind your right thigh. Pull your right thigh towards your head, feeling the stretch in the back of your left hip. Isometrically contract your right thigh away from you for five seconds, and then relax for three seconds.
3. Pull your right thigh toward your head, feeling the new point of maximal stretch in the back of your left hip. Isometrically contract your right thigh away from you for five seconds, and then relax for three seconds.
4. Repeat Step 3, then do passive stretch for ten seconds.
5. Do two sets. Switch sides and repeat.

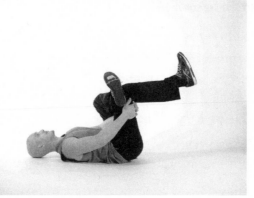

Hip Flexor Stretch

To start: Kneel on the ground with both knees.

1. Move your right leg forward by bringing the right knee up and keeping your right foot on ground. Lean forward to feel the stretch in front of your left hip.
2. Place both forearms below your right thigh to secure maximal stretch. Isometrically contract your left knee into the floor with a low level of force for five seconds, then relax for three seconds.
3. Lean forward to feel the new point of maximal stretch. Isometrically contract your left knee into the floor with a low level of force for five seconds, then relax for three seconds.
4. Repeat Step 3, then do passive stretch for ten seconds.
5. Do two sets. Switch sides and repeat.

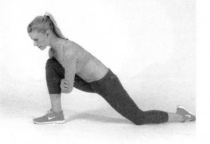

Group 3: Lower Core Exercises

These exercises address the deficiencies in the lower core that can lead to injury. They strengthen the various muscles of the lower core, especially the outer hip muscles, and increase flexibility in the legs.

Clamshells with Resistance Band

To start: Sit down on the ground. Place a resistance band around your thighs just above your knees. Lie on your your left side with left arm supporting your head. Bend knees pointed forward at a 90-degree angle. Keep low back straight.

1. Lift your right knee upwards eight to twelve inches; keep your right foot in place against the left foot.
2. Hold for three seconds, then lower to original position.

Repeat 15 times for one set; complete two sets. Switch to the right side of your body and repeat.

Note: You can also do this exercise with your back up against a wall while lying down on your side. This will help with stability and to prevent arching the lower back.

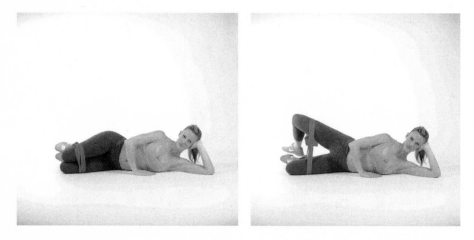

Straight Leg Hip Abduction and Extension with Resistance Band

To start: Sit down on the ground. Place a resistance band just above ankles. Lay on your left side with left arm supporting your head.

1. Lift right leg upward to 35 degrees, keeping the knee straight. Your leg should not be in a straight line with body; it should be angled by 15 degrees behind the body.
2. Hold for three seconds then slowly return to original position.

Repeat 15 times for one set; complete two sets. Switch to the right side of your body and repeat.

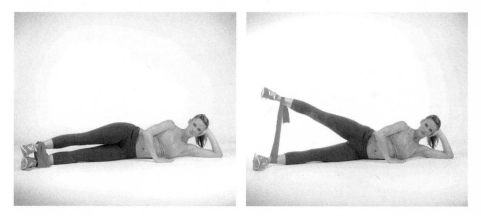

Marching in Place with Resistance Band

To start: Stand with good posture. Place one end of a resistance band around your waist with the other end secured to solid fixture, like a door knob. Step back to create tension in the resistance band.

1. March in place facing the door for 15 seconds, maintaining the tension in the resistance band. Repeat five times.
2. March in place with your right side facing the door for 15 seconds, maintaining the tension in the resistance band. Repeat five times.
3. March in place facing away from the door for 15 seconds. Repeat five times.

4. March in place with your left side facing the door for 15 seconds. Repeat five times.

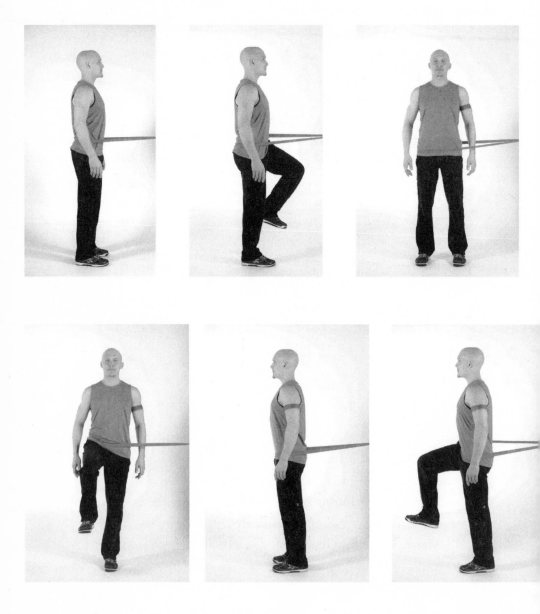

Hamstring Stretch

To start: Lie down on your back. Attach a stretching belt to your right foot.

1. Pull with both hands on the opposite end of the stretch belt, raising your right leg so you feel a stretch in the back of your right thigh.
2. Isometrically contract your hamstring with a low level of force by attempting to bend your knee for five seconds at maximal stretch, then relax for three seconds.
3. Raise your right leg so you feel a new point of maximal stretch in the back of your right thigh. Isometrically contract your hamstring with a low level of force by attempting to bend your knee for five seconds at maximal stretch, then relax for three seconds.
4. Repeat Step 3, then do passive stretch for ten seconds.
5. Do two sets. Switch sides and repeat.

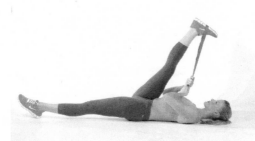

Quadriceps Stretch

To start: Attach a stretch belt to your right foot. Lie down on your stomach on the ground.

1. Pull with both hands the opposite end of the stretch belt, raising your lower leg while bending your knee so you feel a stretch in the front of your thigh.

2. Isometrically contract your quadriceps muscle by attempting to straighten your knee with a low level of force for five seconds at maximal stretch, then relax for three seconds.

3. Raise your lower leg by bending your knee so you feel a new point of maximal stretch in the front of your thigh. Isometrically contract your quadriceps by attempting to straighten your knee with a mild force for five seconds at maximal stretch, then relax for three seconds.

4. Repeat Step 3, then do a passive stretch for ten seconds.

5. Do two sets. Switch sides and repeat.

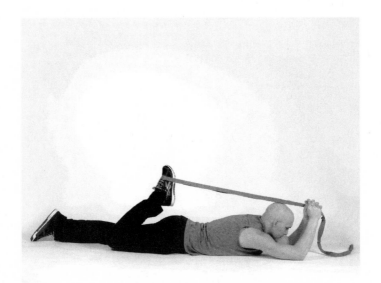

Gastrocnemius Stretch

To start: Place hands on floor, slightly wider than shoulder width apart. Extend legs behind with toes on the floor. Arms are fully extended.

1. Place right foot on top of left foot.
2. Lean back, allowing the left ankle to passively bend, and maintain a straight left knee, creating a stretch in the calf. Isometrically contract the ball of your left foot into the floor with a low level of force for five seconds, then relax for three seconds.
3. Lean back, allowing the left ankle to passively bend, and maintain straight left knee, feeling the new point of maximal stretch in the calf. Isometrically contract the ball of your left foot into the floor with a low level of force for five seconds, then relax for three seconds.
4. Repeat Step 3, then do a passive stretch for ten seconds.
5. Do two sets. Switch to the left foot on top of the right foot, then repeat.

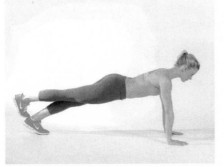

Soleus Stretch

To start: Place hands on floor, slightly wider than shoulder width apart. Extend legs behind with toes on the floor. Arms are fully extended.

1. Place left foot on top of right foot.
2. Lean back, allowing the right ankle to passively bend, and bend right knee slightly (15 degrees), creating a stretch in the

calf. Isometrically contract the ball of your right foot into the floor with a low level of force for five seconds, then relax for three seconds.

3. Lean back, allowing the right ankle to passively bend, and bend right knee slightly (15 degrees) feeling the new point of maximal stretch in the calf. Isometrically contract the ball of your right foot into the floor with a low level of force for five seconds, then relax for three seconds.

4. Repeat Step 3, then do a passive stretch for ten seconds.

5. Do two sets. Switch to the right foot on top of the left foot, then repeat.

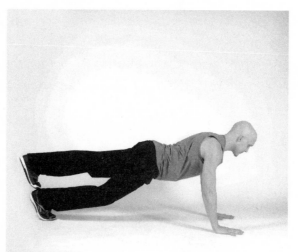

Group 4: Balance Exercises

Proprioception Exercises

To start: Stand with both feet on ground, the left foot placed on top of a stability trainer.

1. Balance on stability trainer on left leg keeping right knee and right hip flexed at 90 degrees each for 90 seconds with eyes open, looking straight ahead.

2. Return to starting position. Switch legs and repeat.

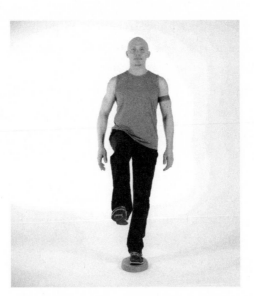

3. Balance on stability trainer on left leg, keeping right knee and right hip flexed for 90 seconds with eyes open, moving head from left to right (shaking head).
4. Return to starting position. Switch legs and repeat.

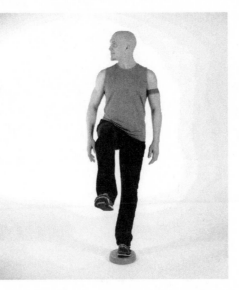

5. Balance on stability trainer on left leg, keeping right knee and right hip flexed at 90 degrees each for 90 seconds, with eyes closed.
6. Return to starting position. Switch legs and repeat.
7. Balance on stability trainer on left leg, keeping right knee and right hip flexed for 90 seconds with eyes closed, moving head from left to right (shaking head).
8. Return to starting position. Switch legs and repeat.

Note: If use of a stability trainer is too advanced, start on a flat surface. Progress to the next exercise in the list once you become proficient. For expert status, bounce a ball at the wall and catch while on one leg (eyes open). Slowly increase velocity.

Time-Out: After Exercise, Don't Sit Down

A physical therapist once taught me to never sit down immediately after exercise. The reason is that your blood vessels are still bringing blood to your muscles, and your heart is still in a revved-up state. It takes time for your body to acclimatize and restore itself to a resting state. Also, when you sit down, your muscles and joints may tighten in a non-optimal position, leading to feeling pain and difficulty moving the next day. Make sure to cool down slowly, allowing your muscles to acclimatize and settle before returning to a full resting state.

When I was working at the Rock 'n' Roll Marathon in San Diego we adopted this information, and as each participant crossed the finish line we would walk them around for an additional one mile "cattle drive." We did this so the athlete's blood would not pool in their legs leading them to feeling light-headed, but also to allow a period for the muscles to start restoring themselves.

Meet Physio/Kinesiologist and Track and Field Decathlete, Joe Hippensteel

Joe Hippensteel is a Physio/Kinesiologist for the Navy SEALs and the owner of Ultimate Human Performance Inc. He teaches advanced training methods and techniques to Navy SEALs and professional athletes in many sports including track and field, baseball, football, and many others. He has a unique perspective on physical therapy because he was a successful athlete before he was a Coach and Physio/Kinesiologist. Joe was a multiple sport athlete, focusing his last three years of college on the decathlon. At five foot eight and 168 pounds, Joe was the smallest Decathlete ever to achieve Division I All-American Honors.

After pulling a hamstring right before two different Olympic trials competitions and having literally over 100 injuries in his twenty-plus years of intense training, Joe focused on developing training techniques that could eliminate and prevent injuries while increasing performance. His unique method of training emphasizes achieving and maintaining a Standard for flexibility called UHP-ROM 24 (or Ultimate Human Performance-Ranges of Motion 24), to create the proper foundation for all athletic movement. The program is dedicated to keeping muscles at their proper physiologic length to maximize efficiency.

For example, he describes his method as the following: "Today, most trainers and coaches believe that only dynamic warm-up should be done before a workout. This is simply not a correct paradigm. Static stretching absolutely needs to be done as part of a four-part warm-up. Static stretching is the only way to get the hyper tense spots out of the muscle to ensure that the athlete can use those fibers before they lock up into a strain. The four parts of a correct warm-up include a general warm-up for blood flow, static stretching to our standard, dynamic movements, and then sport specific movements for your activity. Without static stretching to a standard you are playing with fire."

Joe believes that the best thing athletes can do to prevent injury is to practice flexibility to a standard, which allows complete freedom of movement for all athletic activity. Joe explained his technique: "Virtually every pain and every medical condition to the musculo-skeletal system comes from tight muscles. In this method I've found a neutral point for every range of motion, totaling twenty-four ranges that make the body pain-free. Whether an athlete suffers from arthritis, bulging discs, tendinitis, bursitis, pulled or strained muscles, etc., virtually all these conditions can pretty much go away when you train properly using this flexibility standard. In more than twenty years of intense training, which is really 30,000 hours of research and development, I found almost no other therapy techniques worked until I found a neutral point in each of ranges of motion, which I've now set as a standard." Using this as a base, new levels of endurance, strength, power, and explosiveness can be built without the risk of injury.

"Deficiencies in our ranges of motion standards mean you have a dysfunction which produces pain. For example, take your arms behind you and lift them with assistance to a range that reaches a 7 (out of 10) in pain sensation. Any range of motion less than 120 degrees shows that you probably already have biceps tendonitis. By going through our 'building phase' of flexibility, which may take from one to 100 hours to get to our 'maintenance phase,' you can be out of the 'Danger Zone' and prevent pain and increase performance.

"Through the literature review of those studies I realized that there was no consensus on the duration of stretch, the only criteria studied, in order to increase flexibility. In other words, they haven't really figured out the rules of stretching yet. They only have tested for one criteria. We have concluded 18 criteria that go into our UHP - ROM 24 program. It includes duration of stretch, which muscles to stretch, what order to stretch in, what standard of stretch to achieve, how stretching fits into a four-part warm-up, whether an athlete is in the 'building phase' or the 'maintenance phase,' how injury and genetics fit in, etc. We know that the regimen and sequence of the stretches we developed activate the relaxation response logically and thoroughly for athletic performance without sacrificing strength and/or explosiveness."

Joe's ideas are novel and intriguing because they address the key issue that most athletes face: lack of proper muscle flexibility and ranges of motion which, according to him, is the main reason for pain and injury. Our muscles naturally do not often have the best elasticity and range of motion in order to function efficiently enough to generate the maximal amount of force requited by most athletic events. What's more, a lack of flexibility usually leads to injury. In the context of an overall prehab and rehab program for maintaining peak performance, Joe's standard for flexibility adds what most athletes need to focus on to avoid the potential for injury.

Physical Therapy Specialists

There may be times when you might want to explore treatment options beyond what you can do for yourself. The following are all effective methods that can keep everyday aches and pains athletes experience in check.

- **Acupuncture is part of traditional Chinese medicine.** It is a complete medical system that has many applications. In terms of muscle injury, it can be used to help restore function by unblocking the flow of Qi (pronounced as "Chee"), which is the life force that flows through energy channels in the body. This is accomplished by thoughtfully applying a set of tiny needles in various points in the body. The needles follow a precise map and are determined based on whatever condition the athlete may be suffering from. Acupuncture can be an alternative form of pain control or can be used to help reduce swelling and inflammation. It must always be performed by a professional.
- **Massage therapy** is commonly used to restore physical function by manipulating the soft tissue through stroking and kneading. It can be a very light touch, which is called a flush, and is used to remove toxins from the body. Some elite athletes have this performed on them by a professional after a competition to get the muscles to recover faster. On the other hand, a sports massage is a deeper tissue massage that

is meant to relieve knots in various muscle groups. A deeper massage can also be used to increase flexibility, and is typically done by a professional. However, both of these types of massage can be self-administered if you have the proper tools, like a trigger point massager.

- **Active Release Techniques (ART)** are used where fascial restrictions are released to give you greater range of motion. An ART specialist uses his or her hands, fingers, and elbows to open up restrictions in the body that keep the body misaligned by releasing fascial planes. Normally, fascia is soft and pliable. When it is in a state of dysfunction, it becomes hard and stiff. ART can be a rather painful process, but very effective if used appropriately. For example, runners with tight calves may seek an Active Release Techniques specialist to release their gastrocnemius, soleus, and other calf muscles.

Athletic Trainers

Athletic training encompasses the prevention, diagnosis, and intervention of emergency, acute, and chronic medical conditions involving impairment, functional limitations, and disabilities. True athletic trainers are health care providers who specialize in the prevention, assessment, treatment and rehabilitation of injuries and illnesses. Like a physical therapist, an athletic trainer creates plans for injury prevention. But their most common role is to be ready in case you have an injury. An athletic trainer would typically travel with a team and would be ready for first response. There may be times when an athlete requires assistance from someone else. You may need help to fully stretch or get taped before a competition. If you can't take on the responsibility of being your own first responder, you can easily pass this role to a spouse, partner, or friend.

When I was at the US Olympic Training Center, I once saw a high level swimmer holding the sides of his chest in pain, and an athletic trainer used a Graston tool on him. This instrument looked like something medieval, and the trainer seemed to be raking the athlete with it.

He moved very fast, and the treatment lasted a good minute or two. When the athlete got up, I immediately noticed that his range of motion had vastly increased.

The Graston tool is used to get out muscular tension or adhesions in the muscles so that the fascial planes of the muscles can move back and forth with ease. Swimmers tend to use their *latissimus dorsi* muscles—those found in the middle and low back that attach to your upper arms close to your shoulders—very intensely. Those tend to get pretty tight pretty quickly. But the key was that the swimmer couldn't do this by himself. He needed the help of somebody else. This athletic trainer was instrumental to his success. This therapy was something that he needed in order to have the proper range of motion to create the forces required to get in the pool to win at the Olympics.

Emergency First Aid

An athletic trainer is prepared for any emergency—not unlike the hero of one of my favorite 1980's TV show, *MacGyver*. You can also be prepared for any injury so that you can react appropriately in emergency situations.

The Step Up Your Game First Aid Kit

- **Alcohol pads**—to clean wounds of germs
- **Aloe vera**—for minor burns
- **Band-Aids**—various sizes, to cover cuts or abrasions
- **Blister block**—to cover blisters, especially on the feet
- **Cold pack** (a frozen wet sponge in a ziplock bag makes for a great icepack that won't leak)—to help reduce swelling
- **Emergency whistle**—if alone and/or in danger you can use the whistle to call for help or scare off a wild animal
- **Gauze**—to clean wounds and control bleeding
- **Gummy bears**—in case you feel hypoglycemic they provide a quick and easily portable source of simple carbohydrates

- **Hydrocortisone cream**—for minor burns, external allergic reactions, and insect bites
- **Kinesio tape**—provides support for joints
- **Meat tenderizer containing papain and/or bromelain**—to help neutralize bee stings
- **Mobile phone**—always have a means of communication for safety reasons
- **Rubber gloves**—for protection; helps keep other people's germs and bodily fluids/blood off your hands
- **Scissors**—to cut clothing or bandages
- **Splinting material**—a solid piece of plastic with something to secure the limb such as an Ace bandage
- **Tourniquet**—in case of major bleeding can prevent too much blood loss from limb
- **Tweezers**—to remove splinters, insect stingers, or ticks
- **Warm pack**—to help relax tight/spastic muscles

CHAPTER 4
THE TRAINER

If you train hard, you'll not only be hard, you'll be hard to beat.
—Herschel Walker, former NFL player

There are two roles elite athletes can use to get the most out of their workouts: a personal trainer or a strength coach. These people handle similar tasks with a subtle variation. Personal trainers tend to work in health clubs and focus on individuals, while strength and conditioning coaches work primarily with teams. A typical certified personal trainer or strength coach possesses a minimum of a high school diploma. They conduct basic pre-participation health screening assessments, and based on the results select exercise modalities to achieve desired goals. Then they administer fitness programs based on a specific timeline that is designed to enhance muscular strength/ endurance, flexibility, cardiorespiratory fitness, body composition, and/ or any of the motor skill–related components of physical fitness (balance, coordination, power, agility, speed, and reaction time). They monitor client technique and response to exercise, modifying as necessary. Finally, they review results and modify frequency, intensity, time, and duration to improve or maintain the client's fitness level. For the purpose of the book we'll call this role simply *the trainer*.

When I was a ringside physician for the California State Athletic Commission, I was exposed to the world of Mixed Martial Arts (MMA) and witnessed superb strength and condition coaching. I covered my first Ultimate Fighting Championship event in 2006 and got to know a few training coaches—I was amazed at how much went into the athletes' conditioning. I was later invited to Sacramento to a gym owned by Urijah Faber, legendary MMA fighter, to cover a charity amateur MMA event, and got to see firsthand how the athletes trained. During the off-season a morning three-hour session would typically entail a combination of aerobic training, grappling, and kettle bell strength training. The athletes then went off to their "day jobs," only to come back for an evening session that included sparring and a 5–10K run.

The strength and conditioning coach would reconfigure the workouts whenever a competition approached, always keeping in mind each athlete's weight class restrictions. They could match each athlete's will to compete and continually challenge them by varying the workouts. Without the strength and conditioning coach the athlete's fitness goals would be very difficult, if not impossible, to attain.

Elite athletes are constantly working on improving their stamina and their strength, both of which are required to meet their innate drive to be the best, whether it's for gaining an advantage over an opponent, shaving off a millisecond from their personal best time, keeping a step ahead of their defender, or throwing with more power and consistency. And while elite athletes have the access and resources to have their own trainers, any athlete can take on this role to improve the physical components of their game. By assuming this role, your training will become more efficient as well as more effective. In this chapter I'll walk you through each of the responsibilities of a trainer so that you can make sure you're covering every aspect yourself, including the ultimate workout to enhance performance, based on your chosen sport.

Step 1: Pre-Participation Baseline Screening

Your team physician can and should provide a full physical before you start any exercise program. Once cleared, the following tests are often recommended by trainers. Your physician may be able to perform them, but most likely will refer you to where they can be performed. Or, you can do the following modified versions to set baselines for your own records.

VO2 Max Testing and Lactate Threshold Testing

The VO2 max test determines how efficient your body is using oxygen to fuel your training and competition. The higher the number the better your body is at using oxygen to produce energy. Lactate threshold testing, which is often done where VO2 max testing is available, will help determine your lactate threshold. This is the point while doing aerobic exercise at which your body has maximized its ability to use oxygen to produce energy and starts to use anaerobic means to produce energy, which are not as efficient for aerobic exercise. Using these two methods of testing can determine specific heart rate zones for training.

If you do not have access to getting professionally tested, you can estimate target heart rate range with a calculation; in fact, many heart rate monitors and exercise machines (treadmills, bikes, or elliptical trainers) can calculate this for you. The results are not optimal, but can be useful.

Without access to a machine, use the Karvonen equation to calculating your target heart rate on pages 127–128.

Maximal Strength and Endurance Strength Testing

Maximal strength is defined as the maximal force generated by a specific muscle or muscle group during a single movement. Endurance strength refers to the ability of a muscle group to execute *repeated submaximal contractions* over a period of time to fatigue. These tests are not commonly performed in a physician's office, but can be supervised by a trainer or a physical therapist. On your own, see how many push-ups and abdominal crunches you can do to fatigue to measure endurance strength. I do not recommend doing maximal strength testing on your own due to risk of injury without proper supervision.

Flexibility Testing

A physician can perform general flexibility testing during an orthopedic assessment. At home you can do the sit and reach test to gauge overall flexibility. Sit on a flat surface, legs extended in front of the body, toes pointing up and feet slightly apart. Place a ruler on the ground between your legs. Place one hand on top of the other, and then reach forward. At the point of your greatest stretch, hold for two seconds, and measure how far you have reached beyond the base of your feet. If you have trouble straightening your legs, get a friend to help by holding the knees down.

Body Composition Tests

Body composition testing can determine how much body fat you are carrying, as well as your bone density and muscle mass. This is a good baseline number to have in order to track gains in muscle mass. The gold standard for these measurements is the DEXA scan (yes, it is the same technology that is used to measure bone density, but a different application). You can measure your own body fat any number of ways, like buying a scale that claims to measure your body fat, but it is highly unreliable. The most common tool is skin-fold calipers. You can get tested at most gyms that have trainers. However, the results are only as good as the tester. The test requires the tester to determine the thickness of skin folds at various sites on your body. The measurements are then plugged into an equation to determine your body fat percentage. Ensure that your tester is using the most accurate equation, or you may come up with a result that is misleading.

Once you have your numbers, plug them into the chart below in the "baseline" column. Then, recheck them yourself every three months, and you'll be able to see if you are making progress.

	Baseline	Q1	Q2	Q3	Q4
VO2 Max					
Maximal Strength and Endurance Strength					
Flexibility					
Body Composition					

Step 2: Select Exercises That Expedite Your Goals

Think back to your performance goals, which we created in Chapter 1. How can we accomplish them? Most likely, the answer will be found not by training harder, but by training better.

First, make sure that you are completely knowledgeable about your sport. Do you really know the game, and everything it entails? Do you understand how the equipment works? Do you know if it focuses on upper body movements or lower body movements, and which muscles you need to focus on strengthening? For example, one of my favorite sports is tennis, which turns out to be a lower body game rather than an upper: success is all in the foot work.

Sports in general aren't categorized by what you do at the gym; they are differentiated by which energy system of the body, aerobic or anaerobic, is primarily used. Aerobic means "with oxygen" and refers to the use of oxygen in our body's metabolic or energy-generating processes. Aerobic exercise is any activity that increases your heart rate, and uses oxygen while using large muscle groups. It also is maintained continuously and is rhythmic in nature for a prolonged period of time. Aerobic exercise is centered on endurance activities, such as distance running or cycling, or distance swimming. Marathon running is almost a purely aerobic exercise. Anaerobic means "without oxygen." This type of exercise consists of short, high-intensity activity, where your body's demand for oxygen exceeds the oxygen supply. Anaerobic exercise relies on energy sources that are stored in the muscles. Anaerobic exercise comprises strength-based activities.

Most exercises fall somewhere in-between these extremes and include a combination of aerobic and anaerobic activities. Let's take another look at the Sports Grid, and find your activity. For example, distance running is found in Sector 9: it has the lowest anaerobic demand and the highest aerobic demand; water-skiing in Sector 1 has the highest anaerobic demand and the lowest aerobic demand; boxing like all sports in Sector 3, has both the highest anaerobic and aerobic demands.

Your training will focus on the perfect combination of aerobic and anaerobic exercise that meets the requirements of your sport. For example, a tennis player needs a high aerobic (Aerobic III), low anaerobic (Anaerobic I) training program, which fits the description of all Sector 9 activities. A tennis player needs to increase their endurance capabilities (that's the aerobic part) so that they can perform at the highest level throughout a tournament, not only one or two games. At the same time they need to be strong and muscular, but not as muscular as a high anaerobic athlete, such as a boxer (or any sport in Anaerobic levels II or III).

Level I Aerobic	Level II Aerobic	Level III Aerobic	
Sector 1: low aerobic, high anaerobic	Sector 2: medium aerobic, high anaerobic	Sector 3: high aerobic, high anaerobic	Level III Anaerobic
• Arm-wrestling • Bobsledding • Cheerleading • Climbing • Dance Team • Field events (throwing) • Gymnastics	• Ballroom Dance • Body Building • Cycling- BMX • Downhill Skiing • Mountain Biking • Skateboarding • Snowboarding • Wrestling	• Boxing • Canoeing • CrossFit • Kayaking • Rowing • Speed (Track) Cycling • Speed Skating	

Continued on page 101

Level I Aerobic	Level II Aerobic	Level III Aerobic	
• Judo • Karate • Krav Maga • Luge • Sailing • Water-skiing • Weight Lifting • Windsurfing		• Stair Climbing • Triathlon • Water Polo	
Sector 4: low aerobic, medium anaerobic • Archery • Auto Racing • BASE Jumping • Diving • Equestrian • Fly fishing • Hang Gliding • Motocross	**Sector 5: medium aerobic, medium anaerobic** • Dodgeball • Figure Skating • Football • Field Events (jumping) • Obstacle Racing • Parkour • Paintball • Rugby • Running (Speed-sprint) • Surfing • Synchronized Swimming	**Sector 6: high aerobic, medium anaerobic** • Basketball • Cross-country skiing (skating technique) • Road Cycling • Ice Hockey • Lacrosse • Paddle boarding • Running (5K to 10K) • Street/Roller Hockey • Swimming • Team Handball	**Level II Anaerobic**
Sector 7: low aerobic, low anaerobic • Bocce Ball • Bowling • Cricket	**Sector 8: medium aerobic, low anaerobic** • Baseball • Fencing • Hiking • Softball	**Sector 9: high aerobic, low anaerobic** • Badminton • Cross-country Skiing (classic technique)	**Level I Anaerobic**

Continued on page 102

Level I Aerobic	Level II Aerobic	Level III Aerobic	
• Darts • Golf • Riflery • Scuba Diving • Shuffleboard • Skeet Shooting	• Table Tennis • T-Ball • Volleyball	• Field hockey • Handball • Inline skating • Orienteering • Race Walking • Racquetball • Running (long distance) • Soccer • Squash • Tennis • Ultimate Frisbee	

Step 3: Create Training and Game Day Programs

After taking care of hundreds of athletes participating in dozens of different sports, and at all levels of proficiency, I've found the following exercises to be the cornerstone workout to being a great athlete. Before tackling these two workouts, all athletes must be proficient in the exercises and stretches in Chapter 3. You must have a solid prehab foundation to build upon; otherwise all of the strength and aerobic fitness you are trying to achieve will be based upon a shaky frame, setting yourself up for potential injury, prolonged recovery, and inefficiency in your training program. You will know that you are proficient in these exercises when you can do them all with consistency (two to three times per week), and with minimal effort, over a two-week period. When this happens, you will have developed the necessary muscular strength and proper movement patterns for these prehab exercises and may move on to strength training.

What follows are two separate workouts. The first, a pregame dynamic stretching routine and postgame flexibility routine, covers what you'll do before and after any competition, race, or game and applies to every athlete, no matter their sport. This routine focuses on flexibility and recovery to prevent injury. The second workout, the

Sports Grid training workout, is the more personalized training, and will help you improve both your strength and endurance by working out almost every day.

Pregame Dynamic Stretching Routine

The following warm-up ritual of dynamic stretching should be performed before any game, race, or workout. The body needs to be primed in order for it to perform best. This routine warms up the muscles and introduces a little cardio warm-up, so that you can gradually ease into your game. In the past, trainers would suggest that you "stretch out" before a game. Now we know that it's also important to get the heart rate up, activate or "turn on" key sport specific muscles, and start to sweat so that your body is in a state of readiness.

Shoulder Rotator Cuff Activation with Resistance Band

To start: This exercise requires the same resistance bands mentioned in Chapter 3. Stand in a comfortable position with good posture. Place one end of the resistance band under your right foot and grab the other end of the resistance band with your right hand in front of your shoulder.

1. Place the right arm at 90 degrees to your side and bend elbow 90 degrees.
2. From a full downward position, rotate your arm into full upward position. Make this movement rapidly, one repetition per second.
3. Repeat for thirty seconds, then rest for 15 seconds; repeat two times, then thirty seconds rest. Repeat the routine for a second set.
4. Switch arms and repeat.

Note: You can vary the same sequence to mimic the shoulder movements of your sport by securing the resistance band behind the shoulder, and draping it over your shoulder to work the internal rotators (start in the upward position and move into down position). You can do external and internal rotation at different angles as well; 0 degree shoulder abduction is with your arm at your side, 45 degrees abduction is with your elbow 45 degrees away from your side.

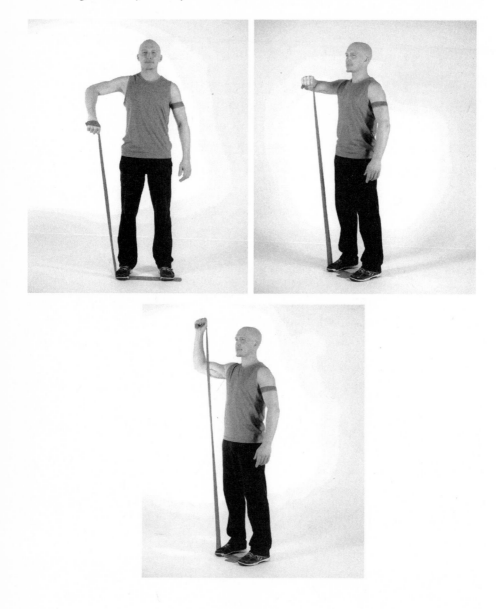

Hip Swings

To start: Stand in a comfortable position with good posture. It is okay to hold onto a wall if needed for balance.

1. Allow the right leg to be loose in the hip. Swing the right leg in front of your body from left to right.
2. Repeat for thirty seconds, then rest for 15 seconds, repeat two times, then thirty seconds rest. Repeat for a second set.
3. Switch legs, then repeat same sequence.
4. Swing right leg forward and backward in a forward kick, then backward kick motion.
5. Repeat for thirty seconds, then rest for 15 seconds; repeat two times, then thirty seconds rest. Repeat for a second set.
6. Switch legs then repeat same sequence.

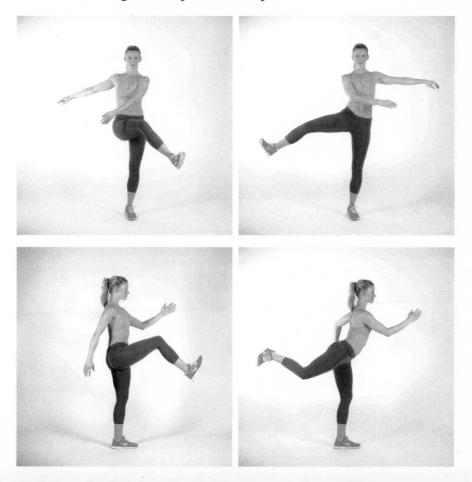

High Kick Alternating Toe Touches ("Frankensteins")

To start: Stand in a comfortable position with good posture. Place both hands out in front of your body at 90 degrees with straight arms.

1. Take right leg and do a straight forward kick and touch left hand.
2. After touching left hand put right foot forward on ground.
3. Take left leg and do straight forward kick and touch right hand.
4. After touching right hand put left foot forward on ground.
5. Keep alternating while walking for thirty seconds, then rest for fifteen seconds, repeat two times, then rest for thirty seconds. Repeat for a second set.

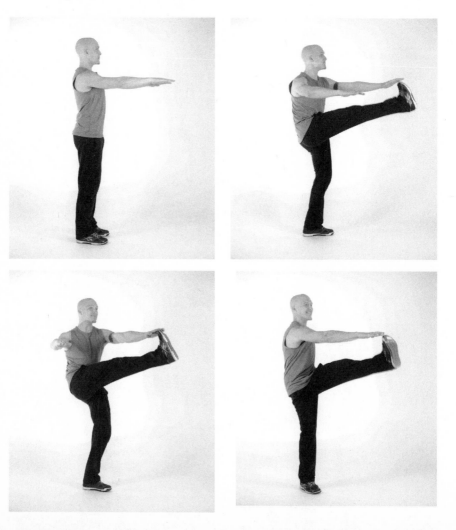

Lunges with Torso Twists

To start: Stand with your hands at the sides of your head with elbows bent to 90 degrees.

1. Step your right leg forward. Flex your hips and knees to form a lunge position.
2. At the bottom of the movement, twist your torso as far right as you can.
3. Hold for one second, return to neutral, and then alternate to other leg.
4. Do for thirty seconds, then rest for fifteen seconds; repeat two times, then thirty seconds rest. Repeat for a second set.

Note: For a more advanced dynamic warm-up, you can do the above movements stepping backward.

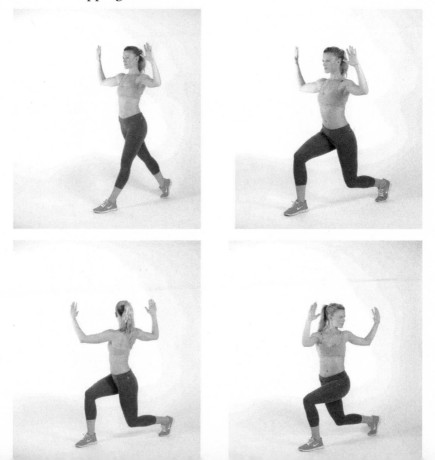

Cariocas

To start: Stand with knees slightly bent with good posture and feet shoulder width apart. Place your arms straight out to the sides with straight elbows.

1. Move your right leg so it crosses over in front of the left leg.
2. Step out with your left leg and bring it behind the right and place it in front of the right. Move your arms in the opposite direction to create a rotation at your waist.
3. Step with the right leg behind the left leg.
4. Repeat for thirty seconds, then rest for fifteen seconds; repeat two times, then thirty seconds rest. Repeat for a second set.
5. Switch to starting with your left leg, then repeat sequence.

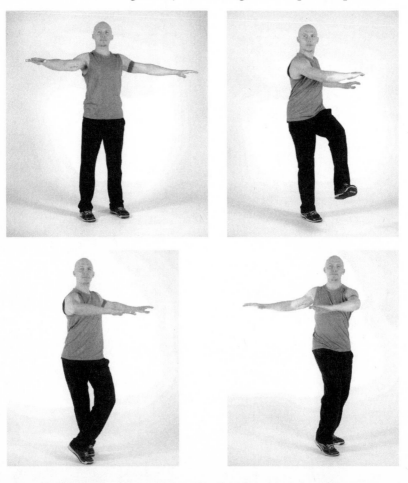

Postgame Flexibility Routine

This short routine allows the body to cool down and restore itself after any physical activity. This period is often referred to as *recovery*. A proper recovery from exercise training is essential for optimal performance and improvement. We know that if the rate of recovery (how quickly you can restore the body after exercise) is improved, you are better able to increase your exercise to the next level without the detrimental effects of overtraining. A full recovery following exercise includes a light snack (see Chapter 5), the following flexibility routine, and later, a good night's sleep.

First, do five minutes of an aerobic workout at minimal effort. This cool down allows the heart to slowly return to its resting state, and can be done by gradually reducing the speed of whatever aerobic means your sport dictates: walk, swim, or bike. Then, complete the following flexibility exercises as described in Chapter 3:

- Chin Tuck
- Levator Scapulae Stretch
- Posterior Shoulder Stretch
- Pectoralis Stretch
- Latissimus Dorsi Stretch
- Lumbar Rotation Stretch
- Piriformis Stretch
- Hip Flexor Stretch
- Hamstring Stretch
- Quadriceps Stretch
- Gastrocnemius Stretch
- Soleus Stretch

The Sports Grid Training Workout

Even though every athlete has different goals, all training programs require three core components—anaerobic conditioning (i.e. strength training), aerobic conditioning, and flexibility. The following workout covers these three core criteria. It is a workout specifically devised so that you can start within your means and ultimately improve your performance.

The following exercises are the most common and effective ones elite athletes use, categorized per level according to the Sports Grid. You can use the following exercises to supplement your protocol if you are already working with a team coach. In a perfect world they should become a regular part of your practices, but if your schedule can't accommodate it, add them in on your own time.

For each level, you will perform all of the exercises in the list consecutively. All athletes, no matter what sport, will start with Level 1 anaerobic and aerobic exercises. If your sport is in Level 1, then stay at that level and increase your difficulty using the 10 Percent Rule, which I explain on page 133. If your sport is in Level 2, you cannot go to Level 2 until you are proficient in the Level 1 exercises. If your sport is Level 3, you cannot go to Level 3 until you are proficient in the Level 2 exercises.

The repetitions and sets listed for each anaerobic exercise are presented as the ideal scenario. For example, if the exercise says to do 15 reps and all you can do is 10, then stay with 10 until you find them to be too easy, and then increase the reps by 10 percent per week. This gradual increase allows enough time to develop strength and coordination of each exercise while minimizing overtraining (breaking down muscles without allow proper time for recovery). Once you reach the ideal scenario, proceed to the next level. The same process applies to the aerobic workout: if the ideal scenario is listed as twenty minutes at a certain effort level and all you can do is ten minutes, stay at ten minutes for one week. Then you can increase by 10 percent per week, which is one additional minute per week.

Level 1 Anaerobic Exercises

These exercises do not require any equipment. They use the body's weight as resistance for strength training.

Burpees

To start: Stand with bent knees and back bent forward in a crouch position, with fingertips of both hands touching the ground.

1. Kick your feet back and place both hands on the ground in a push-up position.
2. Perform a push-up by bending both elbows to 90 degrees or touching your chest to the ground.
3. Push up and immediately return to the start position.
4. Jump up with hands in the air reaching for the sky.
5. Return to start position.
6. Repeat 15 times, then repeat the set again for a total of two sets.

Note: Move as fast as you can, but focus on form and balance.

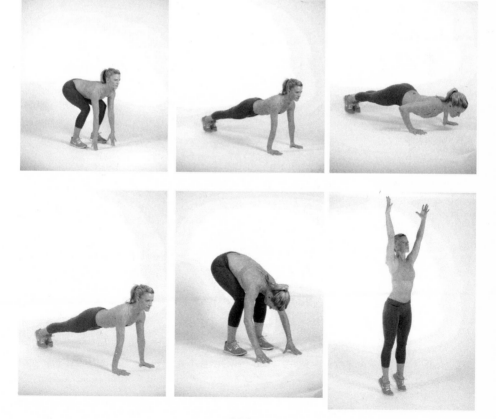

Forward Plank

To start: Rest on your forearms and toes in a push-up position. Keep your body as straight as a plank of wood.

1. Hold this position for fifteen seconds, then take a five-second rest. Repeat five times.

Variation: *Side Plank:* Rest on left forearm and on side of left foot in plank position. Hold this position for fifteen seconds, then take five-second rest. Repeat five times.

Note: The goal is to work up to a continual plank in all directions for thirty seconds. Increase by five seconds per week if possible.

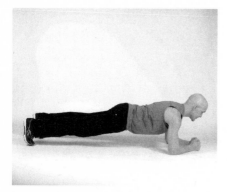
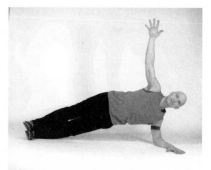

Reverse Plank

To start: Sit on the floor with both legs straight in front of you.

1. Place your hands to the side and behind your hips two to three inches.
2. Lift your body up on your hands while keeping your heels on the floor, body in a straight position.
3. Maintain this position for fifteen seconds, with five-second breaks. Repeat five times.

Note: The goal is to work up to a continual reverse plank for thirty seconds. Increase by five seconds per week if possible.

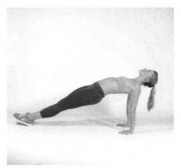

Prisoner Squat

To start: Stand with good posture and interlace your hands behind the back of your head. Make sure to push your elbows back and chest forward.

1. Slowly bend your hips and knees and lower your body to a squatting position while keeping your back neutral (do not arch your back).
2. Return to the start position.
3. Repeat 15 times, then repeat the set again for a total of two sets.

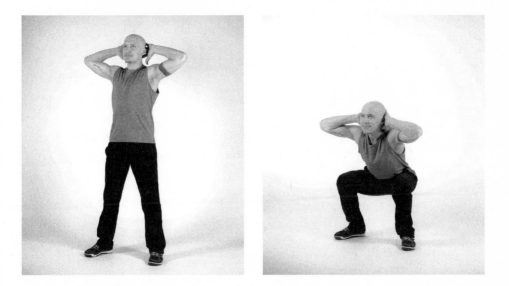

Multidirectional Lunges

To start: Stand in comfortable position with good posture. Place hands on your hips.

1. Lunge forward with right leg forward until the knee and hip are at 90 degrees.
2. Hold for three seconds, then return to start position.
3. The next lunge with be at a 45-degree angle.
4. The next lunge will be directly to the right side.
5. The next lunge will be directly behind at a 45-degree angle.
6. The next lunge will be directly behind.
7. Switch to the left leg and repeat sequence on left side.
8. Repeat both leg sequences three times.

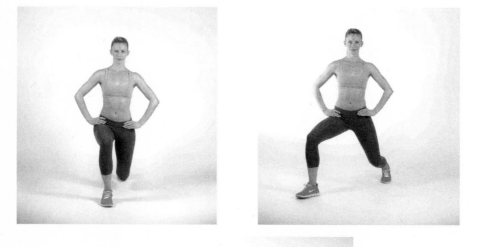

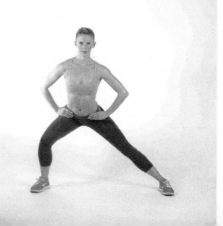

Level 2 Anaerobic Exercises

Level 2 exercises require a medicine ball. This is a weighted ball that can be used for doing a wide range of exercises to improve fitness, strength, and coordination. It can be made of leather, nylon, vinyl, rubber, polyurethane and other materials, and it comes in many different weights, ranging from two pounds to twenty-five pounds. The standard medicine ball has a diameter of fourteen inches.

Ax Chop with Bounce

To start: Stand comfortably with good posture and feet shoulder width apart. Hold the medicine ball with both hands.

1. Raise the medicine ball overhead to the left by flexing your shoulders forward.
2. Hold for three seconds.
3. With explosive movement move the ball toward the right waist while raising the right knee to 90 degrees and twisting at waist.
4. Bounce the ball on the floor while in this tucked position and catch it.
5. Return to starting position.
6. Repeat 15 times, then repeat the set again for a total of two sets.
7. Switch to opposite side then repeat sequence.

Note: If you are not able to bounce the ball and catch it, the medicine ball may be too heavy for you. Pick a lighter medicine ball.

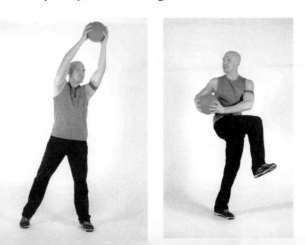

Medicine Ball Crunches with Bounce

To start: Sit on the ground with feet in front. Hold the medicine ball with both hands.

1. Flex at the waist to 30 degrees and twist to do a crunch while keeping both feet about six inches in the air. Kick the left leg out while twisting left.
2. At the twist bounce the medicine ball on your left side onto the floor, and then catch it.
3. Twist to the right side and kick out right leg, then bounce ball on the right side, then catch it.
4. Repeat 15 times, then repeat the set again for a total of two sets.

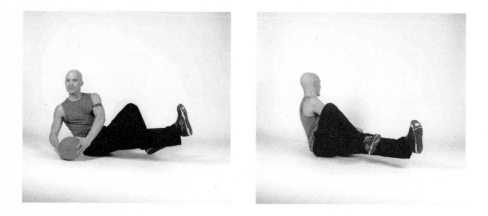

Medicine Ball Thrusters

To start: Stand in a comfortable position with feet shoulder width apart holding medicine ball at chest height.

1. Bend into a squat position and bounce ball on the floor.
2. Catch the ball, then stand up and throw ball up in the air while jumping.
3. Catch the ball and return to starting position.
4. Repeat 15 times, then repeat the set again for a total of two sets.

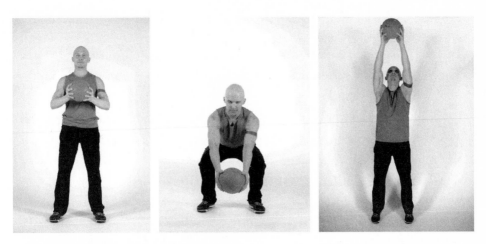

Cossack Squat with Medicine Ball

To start: Stand in comfortable position with feet shoulder width apart holding medicine ball at chest height in front of your body with arms straight.

1. Bend the right knee while leaning right until you get into a squat position on the right side with a straight left leg. Keep your back in a neutral position.
2. Hold three seconds. Return to start position.
3. Repeat on your left side.
4. Repeat 15 times, alternating sides, then repeat the set again for a total of two sets.

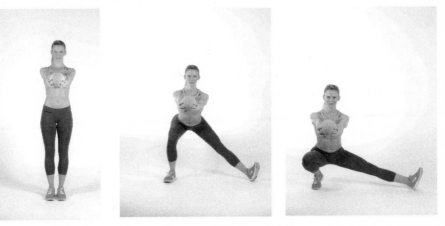

Medicine Ball Uneven Push-Up

To start: Kneel down with the medicine ball in left hand.

1. Lay down into a push-up position, keeping the medicine ball in your left hand.
2. While keeping your back straight, lower your upper body until your elbows reach 90 degrees. Hold for three seconds.
3. Push up to starting position.
4. Roll ball to right hand and catch it. Repeat motions on the right side.
5. Repeat 15 times, alternating sides, then repeat the set again for a total of two sets.

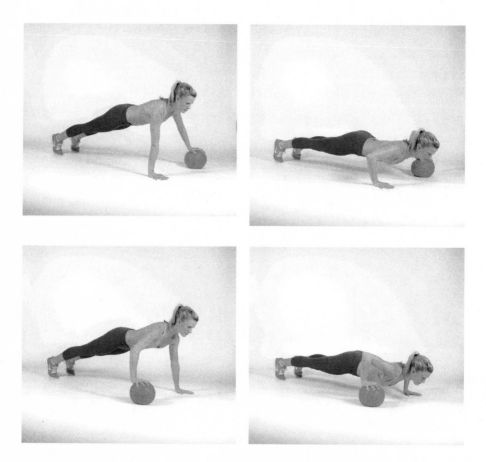

Level III Anaerobic Exercises

These exercises feature the stability ball mentioned in Chapter 3. They are harder than Level 2 exercises because they incorporate balance. They also focus on strengthening the back. These exercises are divided into upper and lower body movements: at Level 3 anaerobic demand is very high, and it's important to strategically target your training based on your sport. For example, if you row, choose upper body exercises; if you ski, work on lower body exercises. If your sport focuses on both upper and lower body, such as water polo, judo, karate, or body building, alternate between upper and lower body exercises.

Level 3 Upper Body

Stability Ball Push-Up Plus

To start: Kneel on floor with stability ball in front of you. Put both hands on ball and straighten body to push-up position with arms straight.
1. Lower upper body until chest touches ball. Hold for three seconds.
2. Push up to starting position.
3. Push upper back upward bringing shoulder blades apart. Hold for three seconds.
4. Return to starting position.
5. Repeat 15 times, then repeat the set again for a total of two sets.

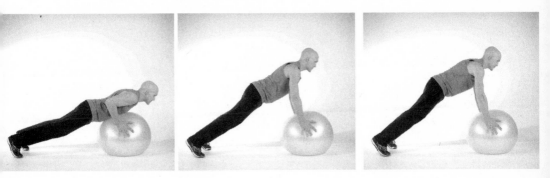

Stability Ball Stir the Pot

To start: With stability ball in front of you, place both forearms on the ball with a straight back and feet on the floor.

1. Move your forearms in a clockwise motion while maintaining a plank position until you reach the starting position. It should take three seconds.
2. Repeat 15 times, then repeat the set again for a total of two sets.
3. Move your forearms in a counter-clockwise motion while maintaining a plank position until you reach the starting position. It should take three seconds.
4. Repeat 15 times, then repeat the set again for a total of two sets.

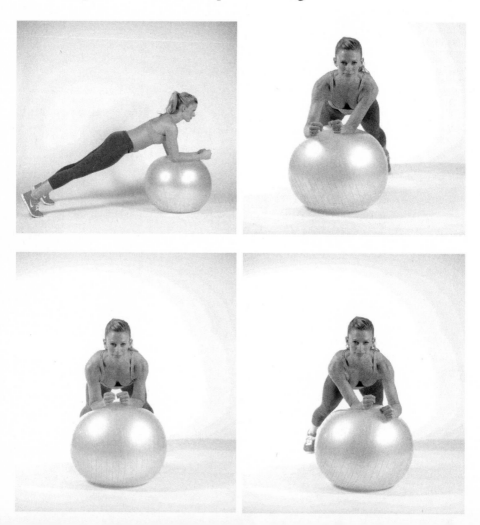

Bridge T Fall Off

To start: Sit on a stability ball, then roll the ball under your back until the center of the ball is at the middle of your upper back. Place your feet flat on the ground so that your body and thighs are parallel to the ground.

1. Slowly shift your weight to the right: the ball should roll under your triceps. Hold for three seconds.
2. Slowly return to the position where the ball is centered on your spine.
3. Slowly shift your weight to the left: the ball should roll under your triceps. Hold for three seconds.
4. Slowly return to the position where the ball is centered on your spine.
5. Repeat 15 times, then repeat the set again for a total of two sets.

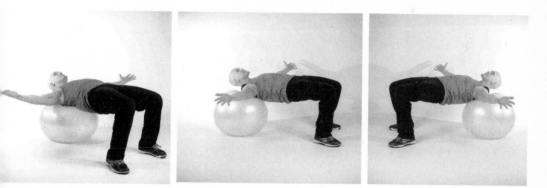

Reverse Balance Push-Up

To start: Lie across the stability ball. Roll the front of your torso on the ball until your hands are on the floor with straight arms in front of the ball and your feet are on top of the ball.

1. Lower your upper body until your elbows are at 90 degrees. Hold for three seconds.
2. Raise your body to the starting position with straight elbows.

3. Repeat 15 times, then repeat the set again for a total of two sets.

Note: If it is too difficult to maintain balance on the ball, place the ball against a wall to help stabilize it. It is also possible to have someone else hold the ball in place until you become comfortable.

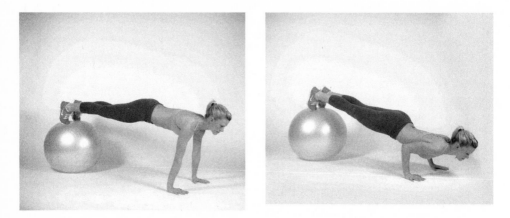

Ball Walk Around with Push-up

To start: Lie across the stability ball. Roll the front of your torso on the ball until your hands are on the floor with arms straight in front of the ball and your feet are on top of the ball.

1. Walk with your hands in a clockwise motion while keeping your feet on the ball. Pause for one second at each "hour." For example, at 12 o'clock, pause for one second, then do a push-up by lowering your upper body until your elbows reach 90 degrees. Hold for three seconds. Then raise your body until it is parallel to the ground. Then advance to 1 o'clock.
2. Complete the entire 12 positions.
3. Repeat the set again for a total of two sets.
4. Repeat sequence counter-clockwise.
5. Repeat the set again for a total of two sets.

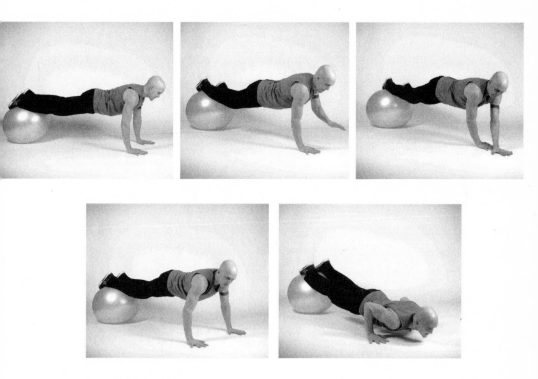

Level 3 Lower Body

Hip Extension and Knee Flexion

To start: Lie on your back with the stability ball under your heels. Lay your arms straight out from your sides.

1. Raise your hips while bending your knees, keeping your feet on the stability ball.
2. Hold for three seconds, then return to the starting position.
3. Repeat 15 times, then repeat the set again for a total of two sets.

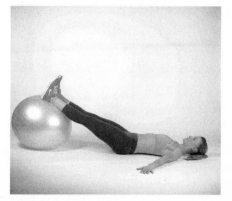
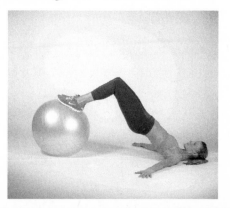

Split Squat

To start: Stand in front of the stability ball. Place the top of your left foot on top of the ball.

1. Step forward with right leg.
2. Bend your right knee to 90 degrees while lowering your body toward the floor without touching the right knee to floor. Hold for three seconds.
3. Return to starting position.
4. Repeat 15 times, and then repeat the set again for a total of two sets.
5. Switch legs, then repeat the sequence 15 times, then repeat the set again for a total of two sets.

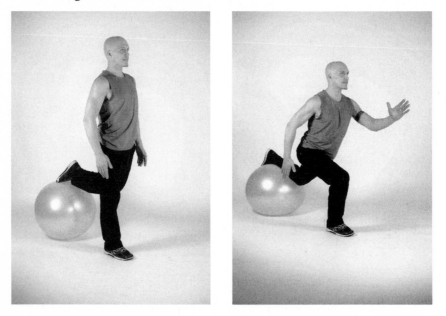

Jackknife on Stability Ball

To start: Lie across the stability ball. Roll the front of your torso on the ball until your hands are on the floor with arms straight in front of the ball and your feet on top of the ball.

1. Extend your hips and arms to keep your body parallel to the floor.

2. Flex your hips while keeping your knees straight, keeping your arms in full extension. The ball will roll as you do this.
3. Hold at the peak jackknife position for three seconds.
4. Repeat 15 times, and then repeat the set again for a total of two sets.

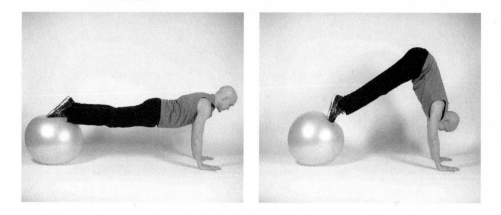

Side Plank with Stability Ball

To start: Lie on your left side with your legs straight. Raise your upper body by leaning on your left elbow.

1. Place your feet, one on top of the other on top of the stability ball while keeping your body straight and parallel to the ground. If it is too difficult, it is okay to stagger your feet.
2. Hold for fifteen seconds. Repeat five times.
3. Lie on right side with leg straight. Raise your upper body by leaning on your right elbow.
4. Place your feet on top of the stability ball while keeping your body straight and parallel to the ground.
5. Hold for fifteen seconds. Repeat five times.

Note: Try to advance this position by holding for thirty seconds, advancing by five seconds per week.

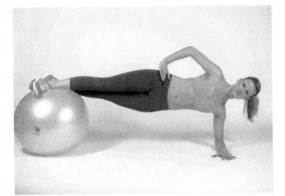

Kneeling Hold and Clock

To start: Place both knees and hands on the stability ball while keeping your toes on the ground.

1. Take your feet off the ground one by one. Maintain this position for fifteen seconds.
2. Move your body in a clockwise fashion, stopping at each hour for three seconds.
3. Complete the twelve hour clock for two sets.
4. Repeat the cycle counter-clockwise in the same sequence.

Variation: For those who find it difficult to maintain balance, keep one leg on the ground while doing the clock sequence, then switch legs.

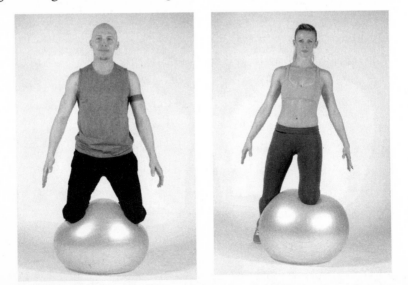

The Sports Grid Aerobic Conditioning Workout

Aerobic exercise is an important component for training any athlete, regardless of where your sport falls on the grid. Every movement in sport requires the use of the cardiovascular system to bring oxygen and glucose to the muscles and remove carbon dioxide and waste from the muscles. The higher the aerobic demand, the more efficient your cardiovascular system needs to work.

Aerobic exercise can take a virtually unlimited number of forms. It includes any activity that increases heart rate and oxygen uptake for a prolonged time period, such as running, swimming, bicycling, rowing, stair climbing, jumping rope, or cross-country skiing. Choose an aerobic conditioning exercise that most closely mimics your sport. For example, baseball or basketball players can choose running to step up their game.

Athletes use their heart rate in relation to a target heart rate to estimate if they are training at the right intensity. Your maximum heart rate, measured in beats per minute (bpm), is determined by using the following equation: 220–age = max heart rate. This is the highest heart rate you can safely achieve. During activity, you want to determine a second goal, which is called your *target training heart rate, or TTHR*. The American College of Sports Medicine (ACSM) recommends a TTHR between 55 and 90 percent of maximum heart rate for most individuals.

The most accurate way to calculate your target heart rate is the Karvonen Method because it factors in your resting heart rate, which is another indicator of your level of fitness. To determine your resting heart rate (HRrest), take your pulse when you are at rest: awake but lying down. The best way to do this is to check it three mornings in a row just after waking up. Add all of them together and divide by three to get your average HRrest. The lower your resting heart rate is the more fit you are. Typical resting heart rates in men are in the 60 to 80 bpm range. Conditioned athletes have resting heart rates below 60 bpm. Here is an example that will help you calculate your target heart rate training zone based on your resting heart rate.

$$TTHR = (HRmax - HRrest) \text{ x } (Training Range \%) + HRrest$$

Here's an example of a fifty-year-old man with a HRmax of 170 (220–50=170) and a HRrest of 60. You can see that he needs to train at a heart rate somewhere between 126 bpm and 154 bpm to be in the optimal training zone:

Target Training Heart Rate = 60% intensity: (170–60) x (0.60) + 60 = 126 bpm
Training Heart Rate = 85% intensity: (170–60) x (0.85) + 60 = 154 bpm

These target heart rates are important to know, but continuously checking heart rates during exercise can be difficult unless you are plugged into an exercise machine such as a treadmill, stair climber, or elliptical trainer, or are wearing a heart rate monitor. Instead, I recommend that you track your progress via the Talk Test. If you can maintain an intensity of exercise at which you can "just barely respond in conversation," or speak a sentence, the intensity is considered safe and appropriate. This corresponds very well to being in your target heart range for aerobic benefit. If you can sing, you are not working hard enough. If you cannot respond in conversation or speak a sentence, then you are working too hard. With that said, you can stay in this range for short bursts to "push the limit" but do not stay there for a prolonged period of time.

The preferred method for aerobic activity is called *aerobic interval training* or the Fartlek Technique. Fartlek means for "speed play" in Swedish. This is a form of conditioning in which the intensity or speed of the exercise varies. For example, if you were to apply the Fartlek principle to running, you would do a five to ten minute warm-up, followed by a steady, high speed for a mile or two, followed by fast walking for about five minutes, then sprint until tired, followed by easy running, then full speed up hill for a hundred yards, followed by fast walking for one minute, and so on. The goal is to have bursts of intense aerobic activity with periods of relative rest in between.

Regardless of what aerobic level your sport is, start easy and increase your level of intensity gradually. All athletes should start at Level 1, which should be considered the aerobic precursor for Level 2, and Level 2 is the precursor for Level 3 aerobic sports. You should peak where your activity is listed in the Sports Grid. You will know when you are ready to move into the next phase of your training when your workouts become too easy. If you move ahead and find that you are not ready, don't get discouraged. Just go back to where you were, and in a week or so you will be able to comfortably move into the next level. All levels start with a five- to ten-minute aerobic warm-up of your chosen activity at 50–60 percent maximum effort (can sing).

During the ramp up to the second interval it may be difficult to gauge your exertion level with the Talk Test, but after a while you will notice the subtle differences between 85, 90, and 95 percent max. If you have a hard time, consider using a heart rate monitor.

Level 1

After the warm-up, start with a five-minute aerobic interval at 70–85 percent max (can barely talk). Continue but lower your intensity to 60 percent max for one minute (can barely sing) "rest" period. Then, ramp up to a second interval for thirty seconds at 85 percent max (cannot talk). Repeat this cycle 15 times (i.e. one cycle equals the "rest period" plus the second interval). After you finish the 15 cycles, do a five-minute interval at 70–85 percent max (can barely talk). Finish off with a ten-minute cool down at 50 percent max (can sing).

Level 2

After the warm-up, start with a ten-minute aerobic interval at 70–85 percent max (can barely talk). Continue but lower your intensity to 60 percent max for one minute (can barely sing) rest period. Then, ramp up to a second interval for thirty seconds at 90 percent max (cannot talk). Repeat this cycle 15 times (i.e. one cycle equals the "rest period" plus the second interval). After you finish the 15 cycles, do a ten-minute interval at 70–85 percent max (can barely talk). Finish off with a ten-minute cool down at 50 percent max (can sing).

Level 3

After the warm-up, start with a twenty-minute aerobic interval at 70–85 percent max (can barely talk). Continue but lower your intensity to 60 percent max for one minute (can barely sing) "rest period." Then, ramp up to a second interval for thirty seconds at 95 percent max (cannot talk). Repeat this cycle 15 times (i.e. one cycle equals the "rest period" plus the second interval). After you finish the 15 cycles, do a twenty-minute interval at 70–85 percent max (can barely talk). Finish off with a ten-minute cool down at 50 percent max (can sing).

Moving Forward

As you progress with your aerobic fitness, start decreasing the rest period (where you can barely sing) between intervals by 10 percent. The rest periods should be:

- Week 1 = 60 seconds
- Week 2 = 54 seconds (10 percent less than week 1)
- Week 3 = 48 seconds (10 percent less than week 2)
- Week 4 = 42 seconds (10 percent less than week 3)
- Week 5 = 36 seconds (10 percent less than week 4)
- Week 6 = 30 seconds (10 percent less than week 5)

Stop at the thirty-second rest period: this should be the minimum rest period. Once this is reached, advance to next level if indicated.

The Flexibility Workout

A flexibility workout should be completed following every anaerobic or aerobic workout. Lots of athletes skimp on this part of their training, but elite athletes recognize its importance for maintaining muscle tone that is not too tight. It also allows their joints to have the ideal range of motion.

I find when cool down flexibility training is done properly your muscles are not as stiff the next day.

A flexibility workout is typically done after an aerobic or anaerobic workout just as it is done during the postgame flexibility routine. Then, complete the following flexibility exercises as described in Chapter 3:

- Chin Tuck
- Levator Scapulae Stretch
- Posterior Shoulder Stretch
- Pectoralis Stretch
- Latissimus Dorsi Stretch
- Lumbar Rotation Stretch
- Piriformis Stretch
- Hip Flexor Stretch
- Hamstring Stretch
- Quadriceps Stretch
- Gastrocnemius Stretch
- Soleus Stretch

The Sports Grid Weekly Training Calendar

This is a two-week schedule that allows for aerobic and anaerobic workouts two to three times per week each, with flexibility training daily. These workouts can be added to your existing routine if they are not currently represented.

	Monday	Tuesday	Wednesday	Thursday	Friday	Saturday or Game Day	Sunday
Week 1	• Dynamic Stretch • Aerobic • Flexibility	• Dynamic Stretch • Anaerobic • Flexibility	• Dynamic Stretch • Aerobic • Flexibility	• Dynamic Stretch • Anaerobic • Flexibility	• Dynamic Stretch • Aerobic • Flexibility	• Dynamic Stretch • Game Day • Flexibility	Rest
Week 2	• Dynamic Stretch • Anaerobic • Flexibility	• Dynamic Stretch • Aerobic • Flexibility	• Dynamic Stretch • Anaerobic • Flexibility	• Dynamic Stretch • Aerobic • Flexibility	• Dynamic Stretch • Anaerobic • Flexibility	• Dynamic Stretch • Game Day • Flexibility	Rest

Meet Gymnast and Coach Wendy Hilliard

Wendy Hilliard has long been a major force in women's sports. She was the first African American to represent the United States on the Rhythmic Gymnastics National Team, and remained on the team for a record setting nine times; serving twice as National Team Captain. In 2008, Wendy was inducted into the USA Gymnastics Hall of Fame. She was a four-time US National Team Coach and was the first African American and gymnast to become the President of the Women's Sports Foundation. Since 1996, Wendy's own nonprofit organization, the Wendy Hilliard Gymnastics Foundation, provides free gymnastics training for inner city youth in NYC. She has served on the executive board of USA Gymnastics and the United States Olympic Committee for gymnastics. Wendy has also been a TV commentator for many sports and gymnastics events, including the Olympic Games. She has performed on numerous television shows and tours with the world's top gymnasts, and also performed on Broadway.

When I sat down to interview Wendy, I asked her about her own athletic pursuits and her training as an international rhythmic gymnast. I asked her specifically which exercises outside of her sport were the most effective in improving her overall skill set. She told me, "I would say ballet. All gymnasts take up a rhythmic activity. When I was younger, I did do some running in the morning just for cardio. I would then do Pilates. That was actually very helpful. I also did Bikram Yoga which was helpful when I was trying to get through injury."

Wendy outlined her typical practice schedules. "When I was an athlete I had two workouts a day. A lot of time I would do gymnastics, and then also do a ballet class, which by itself was an hour and a half. If we were at a training camp, they would also have us walking or a little bit of running. Part of this routine was conditioning, and part of it was to help us watch our weight. Rhythmics is one of those sports where the weight is important. None of the typical activities burned a lot of calories straight out; even when you practice a long time, you're always stopping. Conditioning was also a big part of my training. Gymnastics is a year-round sport, so kids train a lot in summer. When we come back after our summer break when school starts, we do a lot of conditioning, including burpees, touch sprints, and lots of calisthenics. The rhythmic training focuses on strength and flexibility. We also did a lot of jump rope. We do our cardio, not for endurance necessarily but to get our heart rate and energy levels up. A lot of my routines in gymnastics were like a minute and fifteen seconds, or a minute 30, two minutes tops. So while we never had to extend physical fitness for a long time, we had to be able to shoot it up when needed.

"When I was training, the warm-up is part of the flexibility training. To gain more flexibility, you do hard stretching. Then we would do the workout, and then at the end, we would do conditioning. The conditioning helped to become strong enough to do a routine."

Step 4: Monitor Technique and Modify as Necessary

Trainers not only create exercise programs, they know how to modify them for the best results. On this program I suggest that you follow the 10 Percent Rule for both the aerobic and anaerobic workouts: start within your means, and gradually increase each variable—intensity, duration, reps, and surface—by 10 percent per week. For the anaerobic exercises, the variables are repetitions and hold durations; for the aerobic, the variables are duration, intensity, and surface.

The 10 Percent Rule is important because whenever you increase your activity the body needs to acclimatize. Your muscles and even your brain need time to feel comfortable at that level, and only when that occurs can you increase your effort. If we make changes too quickly, then your body may not have adequate time to gain the muscle conditioning you desire. A 10 percent change also minimizes injury: the chance of overstressing the body aerobically or anaerobically is reduced by creating muscle conditioning. Then, the body will be ready to be stressed at the next level but won't be overtaxed. Most injuries are due to training errors—the 10 Percent Rule minimizes this risk.

It's also important to learn how to listen to your body. There are going to be times where your body needs one extra day of rest or a lighter workout in order to fully recover. This can be gauged by your level of soreness. There are also going to be times where the body might not be ready for another 10 percent jump the following week and might only be able to handle 2 percent or 5 percent. Always follow how you feel, unless you are falling well behind your goals or others on your team. If that's the case, you may want to speak with your team physician.

I combine the 10 Percent Rule with another technique that I call *periodization,* which is especially effective when you reach a workout plateau. This occurs when no matter how hard or how often you work out, you just can't seem to progress. Plateaus signal that your workout has worked so well that your body has adapted to it. You need to "shock" or "surprise" your body a bit by periodically giving it a new challenge so that you can continue to make gains. This is true for both anaerobic and aerobic training. Instead of doing the same routine month after month, you change your training program at regular intervals or "periods" to keep your body working harder, while still giving it adequate rest. Periodized training will ensure that you continue to make measurable progress, which will keep you energized and interested in reaching your goals. A frequently cited study conducted at Ball State University has shown that a periodized strength-training program can produce better results than a non-periodized program. The study, which was published in the journal *Medicine & Science in Sports & Exercise* in 2001, showed that the periodized program led to more substantial gains in lean muscle, greater reductions in body fat and more substantial strength gains.

Most often, the reason why athletes get hurt is because they are not using good form/biomechanics. They don't understand the exercise, they try too much too fast, or the exercise requires a fitness level higher than they have achieved, so form is sacrificed in order to just get through the exercise. It is of paramount importance to stick to the prescribed form. Make sure to follow the instructions and model your positioning after the photographs. If you follow the 10 percent per week rule while focusing on proper technique, you'll significantly reduce your risk of injury.

You can monitor your progress by the way you look and feel, and your performance during competition. You can also repeat your baseline testing quarterly to see how you are improving. However, one of the most frustrating parts of athletics is that not everyone will progress at the same rate, or even get the same results, when they follow the identical protocol. In fact, the range can be startlingly broad. This is one of the reasons why we closely monitor our body's response to exercise. If after months of training, you are not able to run farther than before, maybe it is time to change the intensity or frequency of the workouts or try some other type of exercise entirely that your particular body is better suited to.

Meet Triathletes and Trainers Roch Frey and Heather Fuhr

Roch Frey and Heather Fuhr have been involved with triathlons for the past twenty years. They work at Multisports, founded by legendary Paula Newby-Fraser, John Duke, Paul Huddle, and Roch. It is an internationally renowned training center for the world's top triathletes like Heather. With a bachelor's degree in Physical Education, majoring in Coaching, Roch had a wealth of training information to share with me.

I asked Roch what kind of workouts he organizes for his triathletes. He told me, "Heather and I believe in the periodization method of properly building a strong base with aerobic training. There's always some strength training, which is also a little bit of working the aerobic system as well. That gives everybody the foundation to last longer [during their races] and strengthens up the muscles so that they can properly handle all the higher quality workouts that come in the next level of the periodization. On the strength side, I have them doing some type of strength training year-round. As athletes get older it's even more important. Just as they naturally lose strength they can actually net gain."

"One of our pet peeves these days is you see a lot of athletes, and even good athletes, that are trying to train very hard to maximum effort all the time, whatever they are doing, whether it's strength training, whether it's running, whether it's endurance. Their philosophy is like, "Well, if I'm not maxing out, why bother doing it. Is it doing me any good?" While I think that there's a time and a place for that attitude, I just see so many athletes that have taken that track on training and fail, or worse, get injured.

"I rarely have seen any benefit from maxing out when you're doing strength training to the point of complete exhaustion for an endurance athlete. You can get very close, but all I've ever seen is injury problems from that. So I always stress and when I tell somebody to lift heavy; say it's two sets of 10 reps of whatever they're doing, what you should feel like on that second one is that after you finish that tenth rep, that you should be thinking you could do one more. Just barely, but you could do one more. I always try to tell people to hold back from that max complete fatigue repetition. We don't need to shred our muscles; we just need to get them to build up more at an optimal amount without creating too much damage.

"Instead, we try and periodize their normal training along with a maximum effort. I'll take the two together, and I'll start with what I call an adaptation phase, and get anywhere from four to eight weeks depending on the athlete. Just getting them into the groove of swimming, biking, running, plus whatever kind of strength training I have them doing. Then in a second phase, more of what I called an endurance type phase, start to add in more intervals, but not at too high an intensity. Then I try and take everybody into a pretty competitive phase. Whether they're trying for a short race, an hour, or whether they're trying for a five, six, seven, eight-hour race. That's when they will maintain a longer aerobic workout, and obviously longer if they're training for an IRONMAN or a six-hour power race. Shorter if they're training for some sprint race. Then I put them through more of a power phase in their gym strengths-training routine, whatever that is, to top things out. Then go to a very specific competitive phase focusing on their key race and the distance of that race.

"At Multisports we teach our clients to form a core set of exercises that are very similar that you do every time, but two or three should always be different, just to mix things up to stimulate different parts of the body and the muscles that maybe you haven't been using, as well as just simple variety and to kill the boredom from the labor."

I asked Roch how he trains his athletes to monitor their effort. He is also a fan of the Talk Test, and told me, "The talk test is the way to go first. We also try to simplify the heart rates to four key zones that correlate to a perceived effort: easy, moderate, hard, very hard. I tell people it should just barely be getting hard, and then I'll say, 'You should be able to say a sentence or two, rather than just a couple of words here or there.' So, I am trying to give them a couple of different things to think about if one doesn't click in. Definitely, the talk test is always number one.

"Our runners use a monitor when they are going for runs lasting more than twenty minutes. In the middle of the fifteen minutes, we hit start to just see what the average heart rate is, since there is a spike at the end and it will be lower at the beginning. That will give them a good idea of their threshold, if they're going at a hard to very hard effort somewhere in there."

Tools You'll Use

Clothing

The difference between wearing the right gear, or not, is drastic. First, look for workout apparel designed specifically for the type of exercise you'll be doing. All athletic clothing should be lightweight, non-chaffing, and moisture wicking. This type of clothing will reduce the risk of heat exhaustion and make you feel more comfortable as you exercise. Choose clothes with reflective material so that they are visible in the dark or in poorly lit areas if you run or cycle in the morning or evening—black sports clothing with reflective panels is ideal. Invest in the right protective gear as well: if you are going to be in the sun for extended periods of time you need a wide brimmed hat.

According to Jeff Life, MD, PhD, and author of the bestselling diet and fitness book *The Life Plan*, athletes, including runners, wear their shoes far too long. Running in old or worn-out shoes is one of the most common causes of running injuries. Exercise shoes eventually lose shock absorption, cushioning, and stability over time. Continuing to run in worn-out running shoes increases the stress and impact on your legs and joints, which leads to overuse injuries.

The easiest thing you can do to prevent those types of injuries is replace your shoes when they're worn-out. If you've been feeling muscle fatigue, shin splints, or some pain in your joints—especially your knees—you may be wearing shoes that no longer have adequate cushioning. A good rule of thumb is to replace your shoes every 400 to 500 miles, depending on your style, body weight, and the surface on which you exercise. If you weigh less than 175 pounds, you can get new shoes at the upper end of the recommendation. If you are heavier you should consider replacement shoes closer to the 400-mile mark. If you exercise on rough roads, you'll need to replace your shoes sooner. Mark your calendar when you buy a new pair of shoes or, better yet, write the date on the inside of the tongue.

Heart Rate Monitors

The best tool to accurately monitor heart rate during activity is a heart rate monitor. A chest strap model is by far the most common. These units feature two pieces: a transmitter chest strap and a wrist watch receiver. The chest strap picks up the electrical signal your body uses to fire the heart and relays this signal to the wrist watch for display. The chest strap should fit snuggly around the upper chest and must be worn directly on the skin (under all clothing) just below the sternum. Be sure the strap maintains good contact with the skin or the heart rate will not be detected. For women, there are heart rate monitor sports bras that work effectively. The Apple Watch has the most potential to monitor heart rate without the use of a chest strap.

Monitoring Bracelets and Watches

High-tech fitness and activity trackers all share one thing: an accelerometer. The right activity tracker will be based on your individual needs, whether it's step counting, sleep tracking, or 24/7 heart rate tracking. Some have GPS to accurately track running, cycling and swimming with live pace and distances. The Apple Watch is the latest and has the most potential. Other brands worth investing in include Fitbit and Jawbone. Look for features that meet your specific sport's requirements. Ideally, you should be able to pair these devices with apps that can track your progress or provide additional services, such as calorie counting.

Hiring an Expert

There comes a time when an athlete will need to work with a professional trainer. This often occurs when an athlete reaches a performance plateau or is having a difficult time staying on schedule. If you find that your performance goals are not being met, either due to time constraints or difficulty in doing the exercises in the chapter (inability to master proper technique or requiring a spotter), it may be worth investing in a personal trainer for a few sessions.

Personal trainers and strength coaches are not nationally regulated: there are no governing bodies to standardize the training program. However, there are key traits that I believe trainers should have, including proper certification (see the Resources section for the most established organizations). Your trainer should have a full understanding of the physiology of the human body. They should be well versed in the application of exercises to match one's goals. They should have a bachelor's degree in some sort of exercise science. They should have great communication skills and be very attentive when they work with you. They should not be distracted or working with other clients at the same time (unless it's a group class). They should be positive and encouraging, not militant and belittling. They should be committed to your goals, and have a specific method to measure your improvement. They should be flexible enough to accommodate unforeseeable emergencies that may require you to cancel, and be able to get you back on track and not lose sight of your goals. Lastly, any good trainer should be able to explain to you the reason for each exercise that he or she has incorporated into your program/workout.

CHAPTER 5
THE DIETITIAN

Our food should be our medicine and our medicine should be our food.

—Hippocrates

W
e've all heard that having a sound nutrition plan is vital to our wellness. Yet for decades, athletes have been eating whatever they want whenever they want: they believed, as I used to, that they would burn off whatever they ate during play. The poster boy for this was Michael Phelps, who was shown to eat more than 12,000 calories a day during his Olympic training. However, the latest nutritional research is shelving these old ideas and replacing them with a more scientifically measured approach. The truth is, what you eat can really make a difference in your athletic performance, and no one knows this better than today's elite athletes.

The scientific as well as the anecdotal evidence that nutrition plays a vital role in performance is building. For example, Gretchen Reynolds of the *New York Times* reported on one study that upends the carb-loading fad completely. For decades athletes have been taught to follow a diet rich in carbohydrates to fuel exertion, and avoid fatty foods because they are an inefficient fuel source. But in recent years, endurance athletes like marathoners and triathletes have been finding better success following a high-fat diet. One researcher, Jeff Volek, PhD, from the Department of Human Sciences at the Ohio State University, believes that the ideal athletic diet could consist of nearly 85 percent fat and almost no carbohydrates. This extremely fatty diet leads to *ketosis*, where the body creates ketones from the breakdown of fat into fatty acids, and uses these ketones as fuel when the blood does not contain much sugar. Ketones also are believed to reduce inflammation. This theory posits that a high fat diet could both fuel strenuous exercise and aid in workout recovery by reducing inflammation and muscle damage.

Other athletes are changing their eating when it comes to their post workout recovery plans. Clint Wattenberg, Cornell University's coordinator of sports nutrition has been quoted in the *New York Times* as saying, "Fueling recovery is as important as the work you put in." The latest trend is recovering with low-fat chocolate milk, and the research supporting this idea is impressive. The sugar in chocolate milk stimulates muscle and glycogen repair, while the milk's high protein content allows the body to refuel without overconsuming, and continue to build and repair muscle.

Another new strategy is reexamining coffee. Caffeine is a stimulant that has been shown to help with performance, but too much in the bloodstream can disqualify athletes from competition. However, a moderate amount of coffee is now thought to provide a boost of energy that may provide a competitive edge. Coffee and tea are no longer considered to be dehydrating, so you can count them in your daily fluid intake. Another good choice is sports drinks to replace lost sodium while sweating, especially for exercise lasting more than one hour.

Individual athletes are experimenting with specific diets that address real health issues and are seeing great results. For example, in 2012 I was sitting across from John Mann, a USA Water Polo player who was two years into his Olympic training. I noticed immediately that in the twelve months since I had seen him last he had lost a considerable amount of weight. John told me that over the year he had cut out all simple carbohydrates and wheat from his diet, and substituted quinoa instead of rice or pasta. Known for its higher content of fiber, protein, and healthy phytonutrients, quinoa became John's secret weapon for keeping his carbohydrate intake at a much healthier range, while still feeling full and satisfied after each meal.

My patient Marnie had a similar story. She came up from Florida to meet with me because at five foot, two inches she weighed 252 pounds. Even though she always considered herself to be athletic, her weight was becoming an obstacle. She was so overweight that going to the gym was no longer enjoyable: she was embarrassed about the way she looked in gym clothes and felt tired after just a few minutes into her workout. After a full analysis I determined that Marnie had a true sugar addiction, and her blood sugar levels were sky high. I put Marnie on a temporary no simple carbohydrate diet, and over one year she lost sixty pounds. Just like John Mann's experience, a change in her diet allowed her to reach her goals.

Olympian Garrett Weber-Gale won two gold medals in swimming in 2008, and credits nutritional changes for his success. Even though he had always been in incredible shape, Garrett was diagnosed in 2007 with high blood pressure. This forced him to follow a heart-healthy diet and eventually inspired him to start AthleticFoodie.com, a website that helps people understand that tasty food can be healthy. In March 2013 he was one of six invited speakers to talk about the value of good nutrition at the White House.

Elite athletes can make these changes by working with a dietitian. This person will not only create meal plans but monitor their efforts. This role is responsible for providing nutritional guidance so that we can maximize our energy as well as making sure we are meeting the basic nutritional needs the body requires. This includes the proper amounts of micronutrients—vitamins and minerals—as well as the macronutrients—proteins, carbohydrates, and fats.

The role of the dietitian can easily be taken on by any athlete. By following the guidelines in this chapter and customizing them to your specific needs, you can ensure that you are fully taking on this responsibility.

Meet Sport Dietitian Shawn Hueglin

Shawn Hueglin, PhD, RD, CSSD, is a senior sport dietitian with the US Olympic Committee. Her training is in both exercise physiology and nutrition, and she serves as the lead sport dietitian for planning the 2016 Summer Olympic Games in Rio de Janeiro, Brazil. As she says, *"You can't really talk about training, or nutrition without the other."*

Shawn definitely believes that food can be a factor in improving performance. She told me, "Whether it's affecting it positively or negatively… I think it can go both directions. It probably depends a lot on what time frame we're looking at. I think you always have to look at the bigger picture. It's not always the daily meals, but it's what you're taking in before, and then probably during. A lot of that depends on the duration of the events, and then the surrounding food that has been eaten leading up to it. We have to customize it to the needs of the athlete for the duration, the intensity."

When it comes to superfoods, Shawn is less interested in individual foods that can enhance performance, and more interested in getting her Olympic athletes to make big picture eating changes. Ultimately, she believes that making any small change can lead to making bigger, better changes to the way you eat every day. She told me, "While there are some great foods out there, I don't think that the results [from eating any one particular food] are that visible. I can't think of any athlete who I get to eat kale every day, who is seeing some significant changes in performance. But I have seen them stop eating less healthy foods and start eating the kale, or filling their plate with kale and not eating as much of other things that are not that healthy for us. That's when we see changes in body composition because we are able to build a little bit more muscle. So I see it as a sort of domino effect of what might come out of eating superfoods. A big part of my job is to get our athletes to make major shifts, choosing whole grains and complex carbs over desserts and sweets is one area I often recommend athletes focus on. Substituting healthier fats like avocado, olive oil, natural nut butters and nuts, and ground flax instead of cream cheese, butter, fried foods, fattier meats like sausage and bacon. Drinking more water is a daily recommendation for many athletes as well as eating more veggies."

I agree with Shawn's philosophy for two reasons. First, a natural food diet that she describes is not limiting or burdensome to athletes who have time and financial constraints. You can find the right foods that will support your performance at any local supermarket, and your meals can be easy to prepare. For example, when I was at the US Olympic Training Center, I spent time with the chefs who were able to make tasty wholesome foods that didn't require hard-to-find ingredients. What's more, fad diets may redirect you from key nutrients that you definitely need, and while they may lead to weight loss in the short run, they cannot support your activity levels on an ongoing basis.

Shawn shared that at the USOC there is a big push to get athletes to eat foods with vitamin D3 and iron every day. This is to ensure that the athletes are replenishing their diet at performance levels, as compared to average levels. Most people do not get enough vitamin D outside of their diet, and iron is typically utilized during intensive workouts. Both of these essential nutrients therefore need to be replaced. The food that is highest in vitamin D naturally is salmon and swordfish, but milk and orange juice are good choices because they are options that are fortified with vitamin D. Foods high in iron include red meat, lentils, spinach, and oysters.

The Step Up Your Game Essential Eating Instructions

A good nutrition program supports your workouts as well as your training and competition, providing the energy and the basic nutritional requirements the body needs to match the performance that you want.

The Step Up Your Game nutrition plan gives you an easy way to ensure your body gets what it needs. The following is a diet plan that is flexible enough to accommodate the different stages of your training, recovery, and days of competition. It provides additional snacks for heavy training days, and takes into account the macronutrient percentage of carbohydrate, protein, and fat specific for your sport.

This is a maintenance rather than a weight loss program, and focuses on clean foods that support cardiovascular health. I've found that my elite athletes perform best when they meet and exceed the best recommendations for cardiovascular prevention. I've also found that maintaining the right macronutrient ratio is the secret to good nutrition, and is far more important than being a slave to counting calories or restricting food choices based on fads.

For example, if you are having a hard time gaining muscle despite sticking to a regular exercise training program, you may not be eating enough of the right foods. Protein is the source of the building blocks for muscle, so it is likely that you are not getting enough protein in your diet. Match your protein percentage with your sport and then increase it as necessary during your most intense anaerobic training sessions.

However, there's more to feeding an elite athlete than just protein. While others in the CrossFit world might recommend a Paleo, or high protein diet, I've found that athletes don't need that much protein because it will lead to excessive fat formation if it isn't burned as fuel, not to mention that habitual excessive protein intake can lead to kidney damage. Instead, I focus on following an anti-inflammatory diet. Inflammation is a natural process of the immune system to initiate healing by increasing circulation. Increased circulation brings white blood cells to the site of injury or infection in order to repair damage. While some inflammation is beneficial for healing, chronic or excessive inflammation can actually work against you. Chronic inflammation is implicated in various diseases, but for athletes it can also hamper performance. The swelling and water retention involved in inflammation can also irritate nerve endings, contributing to pain, or making pain worse.

An anti-inflammatory diet is one of the best ways to control your natural inflammatory response. This means focusing on fresh vegetables and fruits, whole grains, and anti-inflammatory fats and nuts while limiting processed foods, refined sugars, artificial colors/flavors/sweeteners, and foods that contain trans fatty acids.

Boost your immune system with foods that are high in antioxidants such as fruits and vegetables to help keep your immune system healthy and reduce the amount of free radicals that your body builds up during high-intensity training. Choose the fruits and vegetables with deep colors through and through (not just on the skin) such as blueberries, strawberries, kiwis, oranges, broccoli, carrots, and sweet potatoes.

Grains, along with fruits and vegetables, are going to make up the majority of your carbohydrate intake. Fruits and vegetables are full of vitamins, minerals, antioxidants and fiber. Choose whole grains as opposed to refined grains, which are a better source of complex carbohydrates. Complex carbohydrates will prevent spikes in your blood sugar level, and can replace refined sugars that promote inflammation. Healthy grains include whole wheat, oats, bulgur, and quinoa. Avoid or limit refined carbohydrates such as white bread, pastries, sweets and pastas.

Anti-inflammatory fats include olive oil, coconut oil, avocados, salmon and sardines. Nuts and nut butters such as peanut, almonds, walnuts, sesame seeds, pumpkin seeds and flax are all excellent sources of healthy fats.

Animal proteins can be eaten on an anti-inflammatory diet. When selecting animal protein, choose fish, poultry (especially free-range and organically raised), low-fat beef or lamb, and omega-3 eggs. Animal proteins that are high in fat should be limited because they can promote inflammation. Limit foods that are processed or fried, and higher fat meats like chicken wings, bologna and pastrami.

Many spices reduce inflammation. Some great examples are turmeric, oregano, rosemary, ginger, garlic, cinnamon, and cayenne pepper. You can also eat fermented foods such as kimchi, miso soup, sauerkraut, and yogurt. Fermented foods can help rebuild the immune system by supporting healthy microflora in the gut and to reduce inflammation.

Lastly, make sure you are getting enough water. Water is the lifeline that keeps all of the processes in our body working. Your body is more than 80 percent water and your muscles depend on water to function properly. A dehydrated body cannot train or compete at its peak. Some believe that we need at least eight glasses of water a day, but I don't necessarily follow that. First of all, the general water content of foods also counts; if you are following a diet like this one that is high in fruits and vegetables, you are already taking care of a good amount of your hydration. Base your consumption on thirst, and the color of your urine. When you are well hydrated your urine will be pale, almost colorless. However, if you sweat a lot when you exercise, you'll need to supplement that.

The USOC makes the following additional recommendations to their athletes:

- Try not to go into a training session with an empty fuel tank. Eat a meal three to four hours or a snack one to two hours before exercise.
- Eat to recover. Choose carbohydrate rich foods with some protein within thirty to sixty minutes of finishing a training session to help your body recover faster. Good choices after workouts include: peanut butter sandwich, chocolate milk, or a bowl of cereal with milk or yogurt.
- Sport products including bars, gels, and drinks do have their place in an athlete's eating program. Don't rely too heavily on these products, though, as they can deter achievement of body weight goals and can replace more beneficial calories from whole foods. Use sports products before, during or immediately after practice depending on your sport needs and goals.

Common Food Pitfalls

Elite athletes have systems in place so that their food sources are never a surprise. With careful planning, you can set up a similar program. Here are some of the most common mistakes athletes make when it comes to eating, so you can avoid them:

- **Missing meals:** Missing meals happens because of a lack of planning, such as skipping breakfast if you run out of time in the morning. This leads to erratic glucose levels in the bloodstream, leading to an unpredictable availability of energy to support your activity level. Also, it can lead to overeating at the next meal, causing sluggishness after a big meal.

- **Snacks:** Eating light snacks in-between meals is advised, as long as you are not snacking on junk food or grazing on whatever is around which tends to be processed prepackaged foods or fast food, which are low in nutrients. Poor planning for snacks can leave you feeling full without taking in the right amount of macronutrients, particularly proteins.

- **Eating late:** Eating too late can cause heartburn and can disrupt sleep. Try not to eat a big meal within three to four hours of sleep, which makes the body work overtime on digestion which can disrupt sleep, and therefore disrupt your recovery.

- **Portion control:** The portions we've become accustomed to from restaurants are simply too large. This becomes especially problematic in a buffet situation. When I was at the USOTC all the food was served as an all-you-could-eat buffet and it was difficult for me to control portions and prevent overeating. The athletes had slightly less to worry about because they were burning so many calories.

You can use the following comparisons to approximate different portion sizes:

- ½ cup is the size of a lightbulb
- 1 ounce of cheese is the size of two dice
- 3 ounces of meat or poultry is the size of a deck of cards
- 3 ounces of fish is the size of a checkbook
- 1 cup of pasta or rice (cooked) is the size of a tennis ball
- ½ cup of vegetables is the size of a baseball

- **Rapid eating:** Can lead to eating too many calories. The body's satiety response does not come fast enough to let you know when you are full, which leads to overeating and feeling bloated. Instead, by slowing down and following the prescribed portion sizes below, you can stretch out your meals and digest them better.
- **Comfort eating/junk food:** Foods high in saturated fat, simple sugar, and salt stimulate the reward system of the brain. Some people seek out these foods when they are feeling down or anxious, and then they become difficult to stop eating. I recommend that athletes enjoy comfort foods as a reward, not as therapy. It's okay to eat your favorite comfort foods occasionally, but if it becomes a consistent pattern, it's much healthier to address your down feelings with psychological help.
- **Overeating in an attempt to satisfy an urge for flavor:** According to Eric Braverman, MD, once you get rid of the junk foods that you were relying on for flavor and taste, your brain will not be satisfied unless you eat foods with lots of flavor. If you present your brain with bland foods, it will instruct you to keep eating. But if you cook your meals with lots of spices, you'll be adding lots of flavor without a single calorie. And, your brain will be satisfied with the correct-size portions. In his book, *The Younger (Thinner) You Diet,* Dr. Braverman recommends the following ethnically themed spice combinations. They can be liberally added to baked or broiled chicken, fish, and veggies to create entirely different, flavorful meals:
  - **Asian:** ginger, garlic, and lemongrass
  - **French:** fennel, mustard seed, and bay leaves
  - **Indian:** allspice, turmeric, and saffron
  - **Italian:** oregano, fennel, and garlic
  - **Mexican:** cilantro, cumin, and cayenne
  - **Middle Eastern:** cinnamon, nutmeg, and paprika

Time-Out: When to Eat

I'm a big believer in small meals throughout the day in order to maintain an even blood glucose level. That's why I advocate having three meals with mid-morning and midafternoon snacks.

In general, I don't recommend eating within an hour of training or performing. Your muscles need the blood used in digestion. Eating within an hour of exercise can also cause gastrointestinal (GI) distress and the food in your system will not be fully digested.

You should have some sort of sustenance after every workout. If you have depleted your muscles you'll feel tired and you need to re-energize. In order to maximize restoring the glycogen stores quickly, eating a snack or a small meal thirty to sixty minutes after finishing exercise is key. In the diet below you'll see a variety of 200-calorie snacks that are calibrated for your specific sport sector, each of which provides needed energy for right after your workout or game, followed by eating your regularly scheduled meal.

Eating for Your Exercise Type

Throughout the day, all athletes need to make sure they are getting enough calories. The body needs to support both rest and activity. You can determine your caloric requirements using the Harris Benedict Formula. This will ensure you have the calories you need to avoid running a deficit, when the body will "steal" the required calories from glycogen stores. This is not a good strategy for athletes, because you need those stores in your muscles so that you have it available during your activity. An underfed body will also steal calories from fat stores, which is an inefficient source as it takes time to convert fat to readily usable energy. Lastly, it will pull calories from lean body mass, eating away at muscle and therefore decreasing your strength.

The first step in determining your caloric needs is to calculate your *basal metabolic rate* (BMR), the amount of energy used at complete rest in a twenty-four-hour period.

Basal Metabolic Rate Formula

For Women: BMR = 655 + (4.35 x your weight in pounds) + (4.7 x your height in inches) - (4.7 x your age in years)
For Men: BMR = 66 + (6.23 x your weight in pounds) + (12.7 x your height in inches) - (6.8 x your age in years)

The Harris Benedict Formula

Athletes are typically not eating the right number of calories to support their activity. I've found that while they could be eating too much, it's more likely that they are eating too few calories. To determine your total daily calorie needs, multiply your BMR by the appropriate activity factor, which I've calculated to match the sectors in the Sports Grid. For example, if you are committed to parkour (Sector 5), multiply your BMR by 1.55. The result is your total allotment of calories per day. If you know that you will be having a more intense workout planned for any one day, then modify your caloric intake by using the formula for the next level up, which in this case would be the Sector 6 equation.

- Sector 1 Daily Calories = BMR x 1.725
- Sector 2 Daily Calories = BMR x 1.813
- Sector 3 Daily Calories = BMR x 1.900
- Sector 4 Daily Calories = BMR x 1.463
- Sector 5 Daily Calories = BMR x 1.550
- Sector 6 Daily Calories = BMR x 1.638
- Sector 7 Daily Calories = BMR x 1.200

- Sector 8 Daily Calories = BMR x 1.288
- Sector 9 Daily Calories = BMR x 1.375

Balancing Macronutrients

The second step is to adjust your macronutrient percentages. The percentages for all sectors reflect the American College of Sports Medicine guidelines. The baseline for this diet is for low aerobic, low anaerobic activity, found in Sector 7. For Sector 7, the percentages are 50 percent carbs-20 percent protein-30 percent fat.

The percentage change is marked in each sector. It is important to adhere to these slight adjustments so that your body has the right macronutrient ratio to match the aerobic or anaerobic demand your sport dictates. The sports that require more muscle building will increase protein, while those that are more aerobic will need more carbohydrate. These additions are also modified based on the typical caloric expenditure with each type of exercise.

For example, if your sport is in Sector 8, which requires a greater aerobic expenditure than Sector 7, you are going to need slightly more carbohydrates to support your activity. Sector 8 percentages are 53 percent carbs- 20 percent protein-27 percent fat, so you'll notice the "+3 Carbs" designation. You then go to the Swap Charts, each of which is calibrated to match one of the seven days of the meal plan. Follow the instructions from the "+3 Carbs" category and add/subtract to your meal plan over the course of that day.

Sample nutrition plan for:

Female 5 foot 7 inches, 150 lbs, 32 years old, bowler:

For Women: BMR = 655 + (4.35 x your weight in pounds) + (4.7 x your height in inches) - (4.7 x your age in years)

The BMR equation: 655 + (652) + 315–150= BMR of 1472 kcal

Sector 7 (x 1.200) = 1766 kcal per day (approximately 1800 kcal per day)

Level I Aerobic	Level II Aerobic	Level III Aerobic	
Sector 1: Low Aerobic, High Anaerobic **+6% Protein** • Arm-wrestling • Bobsledding • Cheerleading • Climbing • Dance Team • Field Events (throwing) • Gymnastics • Judo • Karate • Krav Maga • Luge • Sailing • Water skiing • Weight Lifting • Windsurfing	**Sector 2:** Medium Aerobic, High Anaerobic **+3 Carb, +6 Protein** • Ballroom Dance • Body building • Cycling- (BMX) • Downhill Skiing • Mountain Biking • Skateboarding • Snowboarding • Wrestling	**Sector 3:** High Aerobic, High Anaerobic **+6 Carb, +6 Protein** • Boxing • Canoeing • CrossFit • Kayaking • Rowing • Speed Cycling (track) • Speed Skating • Stair Climbing • Triathlon • Water Polo	**Level 3 Anaerobic**
Sector 4: Low Aerobic, Medium Anaerobic **+3% Protein** • Archery • Auto Racing • BASE Jumping • Diving • Equestrian • Fly fishing • Hang Gliding • Motocross	**Sector 5:** Medium Aerobic, Medium Anaerobic **+3 Carb, +3 Protein** • Dodgeball • Figure Skating • Football • Field Events (jumping) • Obstacle Racing • Parkour • Paintball • Rugby • Running (speed-sprint) • Surfing • Synchronized swimming	**Sector 6:** High Aerobic, Medium Anaerobic **+6 Carb, +3 Protein** • Basketball • Cross-country Skiing (skating technique) • Road Cycling • Ice Hockey • Lacrosse • Paddle boarding • Running (5K to 10K) • Street/Roller Hockey • Swimming • Team Handball	**Level 2 Anaerobic**
Sector 7: Low Aerobic, Low Anaerobic • Bocce Ball • Bowling • Cricket • Darts	**Sector 8:** Medium Aerobic, Low Anaerobic **+3 Carb** • Baseball • Fencing • Hiking • Softball	**Sector 9:** High Aerobic, Low Anaerobic **+6 Carb** • Badminton • Cross-country Skiing (classic technique) • Field Hockey	**Level I Anaerobic**

Level I Aerobic	Level II Aerobic	Level III Aerobic	
• Golf • Riflery • Scuba Diving • Shuffleboard • Skeet Shooting	• Table Tennis • T-Ball • Volleyball	• Handball • In-line Skating • Orienteering • Race Walking • Racquetball • Running (long distance) • Soccer • Squash • Tennis • Ultimate Frisbee	

The Elite Athlete Meal Plan

Below is a seven-day menu that meets the minimum athletic requirements. It is based on 1,800 calories a day, the lowest caloric requirements for low anaerobic, low aerobic training for most athletes. This applies directly to Sector 7. If you need more calories per day based on the Harris Benedict Formula, use the snack list calibrated to your sector to increase your caloric intake by 200 calorie increments that can be added to the meals or snacks. Then, balance your macronutrient requirements by following the Sports Grid recommendations and matching them to the Swap Charts.

This diet is a total lifestyle shift that needs to be followed as long as you continue pursuing your athletic activities. Once you master your daily nutrition, you will be able to change your diet according to what your body needs. For example, if you are training for a marathon and want to take twenty minutes off of your time, then you'll need to train harder, and therefore you'll need to eat more calories during your training to fuel your body. You could modify your caloric intake by using the formula for the next level up in the Harris Benedict Equation. If your performance doesn't change, then you are still not meeting your minimum caloric requirements and then you can raise your calories again until you see an improvement in your performance. This may take a week or two to gauge, so follow the plan on a weekly basis before you make further changes.

1,800 Calorie Meal Plan *50% Carbohydrate /20% Protein /30% Fat*

Day 1

Breakfast
1⅓ cup high fiber dry cereal
1 small banana
1 cup low-fat milk
2 tb chopped almonds
Coffee or tea

Lunch:
Turkey Sandwich:
2 slices whole grain bread
Lettuce and tomato
2 oz sliced turkey breast
⅛ of avocado
1 apple
2 cups mixed greens
½ cup garbanzo beans

Salad Dressing:
1 tsp olive oil
Splash of balsamic vinegar

Dinner:
1 large baked sweet potato
1–1½ cups broiled asparagus, salt and pepper
4 oz grilled steak
1 tsp avocado oil drizzled on asparagus
1 pear

Day 2

Breakfast

Breakfast Sandwich:

1 whole-grain English muffin

1 scrambled egg

1 slice turkey bacon

1 oz cheese

1 tsp butter

olive oil spread

¾ cup sliced pineapple

Coffee or tea

Lunch:

Spinach-Quinoa Salad:

1 cup cooked quinoa (tossed in salad)

2 cups spinach

2 oz feta cheese

1 ¼ cup sliced strawberries (tossed in salad)

1 tb balsamic dressing

Dinner:

2 medium baked red new potatoes

1 cup cooked kale

1 tsp olive oil (on kale)

3 oz baked salmon

Lemon (squeeze on salmon)

1 orange

Day 3

Breakfast

Hot Breakfast cereal:

1 cup cooked oatmeal

¾ cup blueberries

2 tsp honey (drizzled on oatmeal)

1 tb ground flaxseeds

1 cup unsweetened almond milk

Coffee or tea

Lunch:

Tuna Pocket:

One whole-wheat pita

Lettuce

Tomato

3 oz. canned tuna

Oil-based mayonnaise

1 tb olive

1 cup baby carrots

2 tb hummus

12 grapes

Dinner:

1 ⅓ cup brown rice

Stir-fry:

2 cups mixed vegetables (broccoli, carrots, cauliflower, peapods)

1 tsp peanut oil

4 oz chicken breast

Teriyaki sauce and fresh ginger for flavoring

Day 4

Breakfast
2 slices whole grain toast
1 ¼ cup sliced strawberries
1 cup Greek low-fat yogurt
1 tb almond butter
Coffee or tea

Lunch:
1 cup bean soup
1 whole grain roll

Apple, Walnut chicken salad:
3 cups mixed baby greens
3 oz grilled chicken breast
1 sliced apple
3 walnuts halves, chopped
2 tsp olive oil and splash of apple cider vinegar

Dinner:
1 ⅓ cup quinoa
1 ½ cup broiled brussel sprouts, salt and pepper
4 oz baked salmon
1 tsp coconut oil, drizzled on brussel sprouts

Day 5

Breakfast

Avocado toast:

2 slices of sprouted grain bread

¼ avocado

Sliced tomato

1 small banana

1 cup unsweetened almond milk

Coffee or tea

Lunch:

Mediterranean Chicken Wrap:

1 whole grain wrap

Romaine lettuce

Tomato

3 oz chicken breast, diced

1 oz feta cheese

1 tb hummus

3 Kalamata olives, pitted

1 large nectarine

Dinner:

1 cup quinoa pasta

Meat Sauce:

3 oz ground turkey

Spaghetti sauce

1 tsp olive oil

1 ½ cups steamed broccoli

2 tb Parmesan cheese

Day 6

Breakfast

Yogurt Parfait:

1 cup low-fat Greek yogurt

⅔ cup granola

1 tb chia seeds

1 tb shredded coconut

1 cup raspberries and blackberries

Lunch:

2 slices vegetable pizza on whole wheat thin crust

2 cups mixed salad greens + 2 tb pomegranate seeds

2 tb olive oil and vinegar dressing

1 mango

Dinner:

Beef Fajitas:

2 whole grain or corn tortillas

Peppers and onions

4 oz beef

Salsa:

2 tb guacamole

½ cup pinto beans

1 cup broiled zucchini

Day 7

Breakfast

Vegetable omelet:

2 eggs

Spinach

1 oz mozzarella cheese

2 slices sprouted grain toast

2 tsp olive oil spread

1 sliced orange

Lunch:

1 cup lentil soup

3 cups kale salad

Dressing:

2 tsp olive oil and squeeze of lemon

3 oz baked salmon

1 ¼ cup strawberries

Dinner:

Turkey Burger:

1 sprouted grain bun

3 oz ground turkey patty

Lettuce

Tomato

Onion

Mustard

2 cups spinach salad

2 tb balsamic dressing

Swapping Macronutrients

In order to keep the macronutrient percentages at their optimal levels, add and subtract these items to each specific day on the meal plan.

Swap Items: Day 1

+3% Carb

+1 orange

-1 tsp avocado oil

+ 6% Carb

-⅔ cups dry cereal

+30 grapes & 1 orange & make banana a large one

+1 cup mixed greens

-1 tsp avocado oil and ⅛ avocado

+3% Pro

+1 oz turkey breast

-1 tsp avocado oil and ⅛ avocado

+6% Pro

-⅓ cup dry cereal

+1 orange

change steak to chicken breast

+3 oz turkey breast

-1 tsp avocado oil & ⅛ avocado

+3% Carb, +3 % Pro

+1 orange

+1 oz turkey breast

-1 tsp avocado oil and ⅛ avocado & 2 tb chopped almonds

+3% Carb, +6% Pro

-⅓ cup dry cereal

+30 grapes and change steak to chicken breast

+3 oz turkey breast

-1 tsp avocado oil and ⅛ avocado and 2 tb chopped almonds

+6% Carb, +3% Pro

-⅔ cup dry cereal

+30 grapes & 1 orange & make banana a large one

+1 cup mixed greens

+1 oz turkey breast

-1 tsp avocado oil and ⅛ avocado and 2 tb chopped almonds and change milk to fat-free

+6% Carb, +6% Pro

-⅔ cup dry cereal

+30 grapes and 1 orange and make banana a large one

+1 cup mixed greens

Change steak to chicken breast

+3 oz turkey breast

-1 tsp avocado oil and ⅛ avocado and 2 tb chopped almonds & change milk to fat-free

Swap Items: Day 2

+3% Carb

+¾ cup pineapple

-1 tsp butter spread

+6% Carb

-⅔ cup quinoa

+¾ cup pineapple & ¾ cup dried apples

+1 cup spinach

-1 tsp butter spread & 1 tsp olive oil

+3% Pro

+1 oz salmon

-1 tsp butter spread & 1 tsp olive oil

+6% Pro

- -⅓ cup quinoa
- +¾ cup pineapple
- +3 ounces chicken breast on quinoa salad
- -1 tsp butter spread and 1 tsp olive oil and turkey bacon

+3% Carb, +3 % Pro

- +¾ cup pineapple
- +1 oz salmon
- -1 tsp butter spread and 1 tsp olive oil and turkey bacon

+3% Carb, +6% Pro

- -⅓ cup quinoa
- +¾ cup pineapple and ¼ cup dried apples
- +3 oz chicken breast on quinoa salad
- -1 tsp butter spread and 1 tsp olive oil and turkey bacon and 1 oz feta cheese

+6% Carb, +3% Pro

- -⅔ cup quinoa
- +¾ cup pineapple and ¾ cup dried apples
- +1 cup spinach
- +1 oz salmon
- -1 tsp butter spread and 1 tsp olive oil and turkey bacon and 1 oz feta cheese

+6% Carb, +6% Pro

- -⅔ cup quinoa
- +¾ cup pineapple and ¾ cup dried apples
- +1 cup spinach
- +3 oz chicken breast on quinoa salad
- -1 tsp butter spread and 1 tsp olive oil and turkey bacon and 1 oz feta cheese

Swap Items: Day 3

+3% Carb

+½ grapefruit

-1 tsp peanut oil

+6% Carb

-½ whole wheat pita & ⅓ cup brown rice

+½ grapefruit and ¾ cup dried apricots

+1 cup celery

-½ cup almond milk and 1 tsp peanut oil

+3% Pro

+1 oz tuna

-½ cup almond milk and 1 tsp peanut oil

+6% Pro

-⅓ cup brown rice

+½ grapefruit

+3 oz tuna

-½ cup almond milk, 1 tsp peanut oil, 1 tb ground flaxseed

+3% Carb, +3 % Pro

+½ grapefruit

+1 oz tuna

-½ cup almond milk & 1 tsp peanut oil

+3% Carb, +6% Pro

-⅓ cup brown rice

+1 grapefruit

+3 oz tuna

-½ cup almond milk, 1 tsp peanut oil, 1 tb ground flaxseed

+6% Carb, +3% Pro

-½ whole wheat pita and ⅓ cup brown rice

+½ grapefruit & ¾ cup dried apricots

+1 cup celery

+1 oz tuna

-½ cup almond milk, 1 tsp peanut oil, 1 tb ground flaxseed

+6% Carb, +6% Pro

-½ whole wheat pita & ⅓ cup brown rice

+½ grapefruit & ¾ cup dried apricots

+1 cup celery

+3 oz tuna

-½ cup almond milk, 1 tsp peanut oil, 1 tb ground flaxseed

Swap Items: Day 4

+ 3% Carb

+¾ cup raspberries

-1 tsp coconut oil

+ 6% Carb

-1 whole grain roll & ⅓ cup quinoa

+¾ cup raspberries & ¾ cup dried pears

½ cup brussel sprouts

-1 tsp olive oil & 1 tsp coconut oil

+3% Pro

+1 oz chicken breast

-1 tsp olive oil & 1 tsp coconut oil

+6% Pro

-1 whole grain roll

+¾ cup raspberries

+3 oz chicken breast

-1 tsp olive oil & 1 tsp coconut oil & 1 tb almond butter

+3% Carb, +3 % Pro

+¾ cup raspberries

+1 oz chicken breast

-1 tsp olive oil & 1 tsp coconut oil & 1 tb almond butter

+3% Carb, + 6% Pro

-1 whole grain roll

+¾ cup raspberries & ¼ cup dried pears

+3 oz chicken breast

-1 tsp olive oil & 1 tsp coconut oil & 1 tb almond butter

Switch low-fat yogurt to nonfat yogurt

+6% Carb, +3% Pro

-1 whole grain roll & ⅓ cup quinoa

+¾ cup raspberries & ¾ cup dried pears

½ cup brussels sprouts

+1 oz chicken breast

-1 tsp olive oil & 1 tsp coconut oil and switch low-fat yogurt to nonfat
yogurt

+6% Carb, +6% Pro

-1 whole grain roll & ⅓ cup quinoa

+¾ cup raspberries & ¾ cup dried pears

½ cup brussels sprouts

+3 oz chicken breast

-1 tsp olive oil & 1 tsp coconut oil, 1 tb almond butter and switch
low-fat yogurt to nonfat yogurt

Swap Items: Day 5

+ 3% Carb

+1 cup watermelon

-⅛ of avocado

+ 6% Carb

-1 slice sprouted grain bread & ⅓ cup quinoa pasta

+2 cups watermelon & make banana a large one & 2 tb dried cranberries

+½ cup steamed broccoli

-⅛ avocado & ½ cup almond milk

+3% Pro

+1 oz chicken

-⅛ avocado & ½ cup almond milk

+6% Pro

-⅓ cup quinoa pasta

+1 cup watermelon

+3 oz chicken

-⅛ avocado, ½ cup almond milk, olives, 1 tsp oil

+3% Carb, +3 % Pro

+1 cup watermelon

+1 oz chicken

-⅛ avocado, ½ cup almond milk, olives

+3% Carb, +6% Pro

-⅓ cup quinoa pasta

+2 cup watermelon

+3 oz chicken

-⅛ avocado, ½ cup almond milk, olives, 1 tsp oil, 2 tb Parmesan

+6% Carb, +3% Pro

-½ cup quinoa pasta & 1 slice sprouted grain bread

+2 cups watermelon & make banana a large one & 2 tb dried cranberries

+½ cup steamed broccoli

+1 oz chicken

-⅛ avocado, ½ cup almond milk, olives, 1 tsp oil, 2 tb Parmesan

+6% Carb, +6% Pro

-½ cup quinoa pasta & 1 slice sprouted grain bread

+2 cups watermelon & make banana a large one & 2 tb dried cranberries

+½ cup steamed broccoli

Change ground turkey to ground turkey breast

+3 oz ground turkey breast

-⅛ avocado, ½ cup almond milk, olives, 1 tsp oil, 2 tb Parmesan

Swap Items: Day 6

+ 3% Carb

+12 cherries

-1 tb shredded coconut

+ 6% Carb

-⅔ cup granola

+12 cherries & ¾ cup dried pears

+1 cup mixed greens

-1 tb shredded coconut & 1 tb olive oil and vinegar dressing

+3% Pro

+1 oz beef

-1 tb shredded coconut & 1 tb olive oil and vinegar dressing

+6% Pro

-⅓ cup granola

+12 cherries

Change beef fajitas to chicken:

+3 oz chicken

-1 tb shredded coconut & 1 tb olive oil and vinegar dressing

+3% Carb, +3 % Pro

+12 cherries

Change beef fajitas to chicken:

+1 oz chicken

-1 tb shredded coconut & 1 tb olive oil and vinegar dressing

+3% Carb, +6% Pro

-⅓ cup granola

+24 cherries

Change beef fajitas to chicken:

+3 oz chicken

-1 tb shredded coconut, 1 tb chia seeds, 1 tb olive oil & vinegar dressing

+6% Carb, +3% Pro

-⅔ cup granola

+12 cherries & ¾ cup dried pears

+1 cup mixed greens

Change beef fajitas to chicken:

+1 oz chicken

-1 tb shredded coconut, 1 tb chia seeds, 1 tb olive oil & vinegar dressing

+6% Carb, +6% Pro

-⅔ cup granola

+12 cherries & ¾ cup dried pears

+1 cup mixed greens

Change beef fajitas to chicken:

+3 oz chicken, 1 tb shredded coconut, 1 tb chia seeds, 1 tb olive oil vinegar

Swap Items: Day 7

+ 3% Carb

+2 tb dried cranberries

-1 tb balsamic dressing

+ 6% Carb

-1 slice sprouted grain bread & ½ cup lentil soup

+2 tb dried cranberries & ¾ cup blueberries & 30 cherries

+1 cup spinach

-1 tb balsamic dressing & 1 tsp olive oil spread

+3% Pro

+1 oz ground turkey

-1 tb balsamic dressing & 1 tsp olive oil spread

+6% Pro

-½ cup lentil soup

+2 tb dried cranberries

+3 oz ground turkey

-1 tb balsamic dressing & 2 tsps olive oil spread & 1 tsp olive oil

+ 3% Carb, + 3 % Pro

+2 tb dried cranberries

+1 oz ground turkey

-1 tb balsamic dressing & 1 tsp olive oil spread & 1 tsp olive oil

+ 3% Carb, + 6% Pro

-½ cup lentil soup

+2 tb dried cranberries & ¾ cup blueberries

+3 oz ground turkey

-1 tb balsamic dressing & 2 tsp olive oil spread & 2 tsp olive oil

+ 6% Carb, + 3% Pro

-1 slice sprouted grain bread & ½ cup lentil soup

+2 tb dried cranberries & ¾ cup blueberries & 30 cherries

+1 cup spinach

+1 oz ground turkey

-1 tb balsamic dressing & 2 tsps olive oil spread & 1 tsp olive oil

+6% Carb, +6% Pro

-1 slice sprouted grain bread & ½ cup lentil soup

+ 2 tb dried cranberries & ¾ cup blueberries & 12 cherries

+1 cup spinach

+3 oz ground turkey

-2 tb balsamic dressing & 2 tsp olive oil spread & 2 tsp olive oil

Vegetarian Protein Substitutions for 3 ounces of Chicken, Beef or Fish
✓ 10 ounces tofu
✓ 1 ½ cups beans or lentils
✓ 1 ½ cups edamame
✓ 6 tablespoons hemp seeds
✓ 3 ounces almonds
✓ ¼ cup seitan
✓ 6 tablespoons almond butter

Step Up Your Game Shakes

One of the best ways to ensure that you are meeting your nutritional requirements is with shakes. My athletes use these shakes as a snack to provide the nutrients and calories necessary.

I start with a good base protein. I like hemp protein because it causes the lowest amount of inflammation. If I'm using the shake as a recovery snack, I might add whey protein, which has some of the same properties found in chocolate milk. Then I always add at least one fruit or some kale. Fruit is a whole food that provides natural sugars and a good source of carbohydrates; the kale is a more complex carbohydrate that also provides fiber. Then I may add some sort of nut—a good source of healthy fat that helps me feel fuller for a longer period of time. I typically choose either almond butter or some whole nut.

Last, I try to add at least one superfood. These have highly concentrated nutrients including antioxidants, polyphenols, flavonoids, minerals, and vitamins. Blueberries, acai, cocoa powder, chia seeds, or flax seeds, and sprouts are some of my favorites. You can also address any specific health concerns you may have per the chart below:

Symptom	Additional Shake Ingredients
Irritability	Saffron, nutmeg, soybean, eggs
Poor sleep	Pumpkin seed
Joint aches	Chia seed, flax seed (omega-3 fatty acid)
Body aches	Pomegranate, ginger

Symptom	Additional Shake Ingredients
Sore throat	Sage
Headache	Coffee
Allergies	Whole grains
Constipation	Fiber: green leafy veggies or add fiber supplement
Bloating, bowel symptoms	Kefir, yogurt
Dry skin	Coconut oil, avocado

200 Calorie Shakes

You can choose one of two shakes per day based on where your sport falls on the Sports Grid. These shakes can be used as snacks. Choose your shake to match your training workout. For example, if are participating in a Sector 5 sport, choose either the Aerobic Level 2 shake on your aerobic workout day, or the Anaerobic Level 2 shake on your strength training day. Or, use the shakes to match your game day's requirements. If your sport requires strength, choose your anaerobic shake, which has a higher percentage of protein. If your sport requires endurance, choose your aerobic shake option which is higher in carbohydrates.

- **Example 1:** You are participating in a Sector 1 sport. Choose either an Aerobic Level 1 or Anaerobic Level 3 shake.
- **Example 2:** You are participating in a Sector 3 sport. Choose either an Aerobic Level 3 or Anaerobic Level 3 shake.
- **Example 3:** You are participating in a Sector 9 sport. Choose either an Aerobic Level 3 or Anaerobic Level 1 shake.

Aerobic Level 1 Shake—carb 50%

¼ cup low-fat 1% milk
½ medium banana
2 teaspoons almond butter
½ cup frozen raspberries
2 teaspoons unflavored hemp seed protein powder
½ cup ice

Aerobic Level 2 Shake—carb 53%

½ cup kale

1 teaspoon hemp powder

2 teaspoons chia seeds

2 ounces orange juice

¼ cup frozen mango

¼ cup frozen strawberries

⅓ cup 2% plain Greek yogurt

½ cup ice

Aerobic Level III Shake—carb 56%

½ cup kale

1 teaspoon hemp powder

2 teaspoons chia seeds

3 ounces 100% orange juice

¼ cup frozen mango

¼ cup frozen strawberries

¼ cup 2% plain Greek yogurt

Anaerobic Level 1 Shake—protein 20%

¼ cup Greek yogurt

1 medium banana

1 ½ tablespoon unsweetened cocoa powder

2 ounces light coconut milk

½ teaspoon vanilla

1 teaspoon hemp protein powder

½ cup ice

Anaerobic Level 2 Shake—protein 23%

¼ cup Greek yogurt

½ medium banana

½ tablespoon unsweetened cocoa powder

3 ounces lite coconut milk

½ teaspoon vanilla

1 teaspoon hemp protein powder

½ cup ice

Anaerobic Level 3 Shake—protein 26%

½ cup kale

1 teaspoon hemp protein powder

2 teaspoon chia seeds

3 ounces orange juice

¼ cup frozen mango

¼ cup frozen strawberries

¼ cup 2% plain Greek yogurt

Additional 200 Calorie Snacks (Pick one check-marked item)			
Aerobic Level I	Aerobic Level II	Aerobic Level III	Anaerobic Level 3
Sector 1: 50% Carb /26% Pro/ 24% Fat	Sector 2: 53% Carb /26%Pro/ 21% Fat	Sector 3: 56% Carb /26% Pro/ 18% Fat	
✓ 1 whole wheat pita + 1 oz roast beef + sliced tomato ✓ **Grilled cheese sandwich:** 1 whole grain English muffin + 1 oz cheese + sliced tomato ✓ 1 cup chocolate milk	✓ 1 cup low-fat Greek yogurt + ¾ cup blackberries ✓ 10–12 whole grain crackers + 1 string cheese + 2 mandarins ✓ 1 cup low-fat milk + ½ banana	✓ 20–25 whole grain crackers + 1 cheese stick ✓ 1 cup dry whole grain cereal + 1 hard-boiled egg ✓ **Grilled cheese:** 2 slices whole grain bread + 1 oz of melted cheese	

Sector 4: 50% Carb /23% Pro/ 27% Fat	Sector 5: 53% Carb /23% Pro/ 24% Fat	Sector 6: 56% Carb /23% Pro/ 21% Fat	Anaerobic Level 2
✓ 30 grapes + 2 ounces sliced turkey ✓ 1 large apple + 1 oz cheese + 1 hard-boiled egg ✓ 1 cup low-fat Greek yogurt + ¾ cup blueberries + 2 tb slivered almonds	✓ 10–12 whole grain crackers + 1 cup baby carrots + 2 tb hummus +¾ cup raspberries ✓ 1 slice whole grain bread + 1 ½ tsp cashew butter + 1¼ cup strawberries ✓ ¼ cup cooked quinoa + 1 tsp olive oil + 1 oz feta cheese + chopped tomatoes	✓ 1 quesadilla: 1 12-inch whole grain tortilla + 1 oz melted cheese ✓ ¾ cup whole grain cereal + 1 cup reduced fat milk ✓ **Turkey sandwich:** 2 slices whole grain bread + 1 oz turkey	
Sector 7: 50% Carb/ 20% Pro/ 30% Fat	Sector 8: 53% Carb/ 20% Pro/ 27% Fat	Sector 9: 56% Carb/ 20% Pro/ 24% Fat	Anaerobic Level 1
✓ One large apple + 1 cheese stick ✓ 1 cup low-fat Greek yogurt + 1 ¼ cup fresh berries ✓ 1 whole grain pita + 1 cup celery + 2 tb hummus	✓ 10–12 whole grain crackers + 1 apple + 8 almonds ✓ 1 slice whole grain bread + 1½ tsp cashew butter + 1 small sliced banana ✓ ¼ cup cooked oatmeal + 3 walnut halves +2 tb raisins	✓ ¼ cup cooked oatmeal + 2 tb dried cranberries + 2 tb slivered almonds ✓ 10–12 whole grain crackers + 12 grapes + 2 tb hummus ✓ 1 slice whole grain toast + 1 ½ tsp peanut butter + 1 sliced pear	

Dietary Quick Fixes

Assess your health after every workout and choose the right foods to re-energize and address how you may be feeling. For example, some of the signs of overtraining are brain fog, muscle soreness, and changes in sleep. These can also occur when you're deprived of certain nutrients.

To quickly resolve the following issues, the go-to foods are:

- **Brain Fog**—Make sure that you are well hydrated. Also, hypoglycemia can cause brain fog—have fresh fruit that is high in natural sugars like grapes. You can also have a caffeinated beverage that is cold, such as iced coffee or iced tea.
- **Muscle Soreness**—Eat foods that are high in antioxidants that reduce inflammation, such as blueberries or pomegranate juice. Eat foods high in omega-3 fatty acids, like omega-3 enriched eggs, add flax seeds to shakes or plain yogurt.
- **Changes in Sleep**—Foods high in tryptophan such as nuts, bananas, and honey. You can also drink chamomile tea to relax.
- **Cramps**—Stay well hydrated and maintain adequate stores of glycogen and sodium. Salted whole wheat pretzels are an excellent choice. Other minerals that will help reduce cramping include potassium found in oranges, bananas, spinach, and potatoes; and magnesium found in dark green leafy veggies, nuts and seeds, fish, soybeans, avocado, bananas, dark chocolate, and yogurt.
- **Short-Term Fatigue**—When you need a quick energy boost look for fruits that are high in simple, natural sugars, like oranges or bananas. A granola bar that contains nut butter or a few nuts is another good option.
- **Long-Term Fatigue**—Increase the proteins and healthy fats in your daily diet. Try adding salmon, avocado, or eggs, and higher fiber carbs like green leafy vegetables.
- **Respiratory and GI Illness**—Probiotics, found in supplements and also yogurt and other fermented foods like kimchi and sauerkraut, can help anyone develop better intestinal health. What's more, the

latest studies show that changing gut flora or bacteria can affect your athletic performance. Most probiotics contain lactobacilli and bifidobacteria. While there is not a strong consensus on the amount you should take, if you choose to use a supplement, select one that is refrigerated with a minimum of 10 billion CFUs, which should be clearly marked on the bottle.

Dietitians Track What You Eat

When dietitians work with elite athletes, they teach them to create detailed records of their food intake and correlate it to their performance. You can do the same. Record your food choices each day, for every meal, in a food log, including the modifications you make. By tracking what you eat you are creating a data set to determine if your nutrition is helping you meet your goals, and whether you are eating enough—or too much—for your activity level. You'll also be able to track if your levels of fatigue and energy are improving; also if your mood as well as your overall health are improving.

After you have kept your workout and nutrition logs for a few weeks you can begin to analyze the information that you have gathered. You may find that specific foods affect the way you feel, either positively or negatively. Some people have a real intolerance to certain foods. This is completely different from a food allergy.

Some people may be lactose intolerant or intolerant to certain preservatives or sulfites. One of the more popular trends is going gluten free as a response to a food intolerance. If certain foods make you feel bloated or otherwise uncomfortable after eating, you can further modify your plan to eliminate those foods. Some people find that once they remove the offending food from their diet, just like John Mann did, their performance dramatically improves.

It's easier than ever to track what you eat. There are plenty of high tech apps that can keep you on track using your smartphone or computer. You can also use the low-tech log below, which acts as a weekly food journal.

You can download this form from my website (www.stepupyourgame.nyc) and keep them in a binder to monitor your progress.

For the category marked "overall health assessment," write in how you feel at the end of each day. Ask yourself the following questions, and write down any negative answers:

1. Am I progressing toward my stated goals?
2. Are my energy levels good?
3. Do I feel like I'm recovering after my workouts? Is the meal plan supporting my workouts?
4. Is my mood consistent throughout the day?

Week 1	Monday	Tuesday	Wednesday	Thursday	Friday	Saturday	Sunday
Breakfast							
Snack							
Lunch							
Snack							
Dinner							
Additions/ Modifications							
Overall Health Assessment							

Finding the Right Dietitian

You may need to hire a professional dietitian if you are having difficulty with the meal plan in this chapter, or if you have special dietary requirements related to a medical condition. A dietitian can work with this meal plan and modify it for you so that it is safe to follow, or make other, more specialized recommendations that take your personal health situation into consideration.

A dietitian is a licensed, board certified, regulated professional. While a nutritionist can also be well trained, they are not licensed or regulated. If you need to hire one, look for someone who is knowledgeable in sports performance: seeing a dietitian who is a renal (kidney) specialist for example is not going to help you if that is not your issue. I would also recommend that any dietitian you hire should have a minimum two years of experience working with at least competitive recreational athletes, and should have a master's degree or higher in nutrition or exercise science. A dietitian should always carry liability insurance, be willing to enter into a consulting contract, and be able to provide references.

A good dietitian will not promote fad diets, or prescribe a generic eating program to every client. Make sure that they are taking your unique needs into account. They should also be sensitive to cultural eating styles or religious observances. They should be able to create both long- and short-term goals for you that are related to the goals you created in Chapter 1. Most importantly, they should not be a vehicle to sell you a supplement line. I strongly believe that you can get almost all of your nutritional requirements from whole foods, and I do not believe any athletes need supplements in order to gain a nutritional advantage for performance.

One great resource is the Academy of Nutrition and Dietetics (AND). Their website, www.eatright.org, allows you to plug in your zip code and find a registered dietitian near you. For those who want to use a sport dietitian only (which is what I prefer) refine the search for sport nutrition.

CHAPTER 6
THE COACH

Coach players like they are all game-winning players.
—*Rick Pitino*

Elite athletes rely on their coaches to help them reach their goals, whether they are connected to a specific increase in performance, or to win a game, a season, or a championship. The coach's role straddles both the mental aspects of the game as well as the physical, and the best ones are both motivating and informative. Their guidance is physical, psychological, and tactical.

They provide a clear set of directions so that you know what's necessary to win, and what kind of commitment it takes to get you to the next level. They will also teach you the ins and outs of your game, and make sure you understand all of the rules, correct your positioning, and teach you specific techniques so that you can succeed.

You may already have a coach that works with your team. In this chapter, you'll learn about the coach's perspective, and how you can get the most of out of this relationship by having a better understanding of his or her motivations. If you don't have a coach, you can take on this role yourself. But don't be fooled: taking on this role is not going to make your practices any easier. However, you may find that you are much happier during practice and game days because you will learn to manage your time and training better. Once you have a solid understanding of what is expected of you, it will be much easier to break through the obstacles that are holding you back. What's more, you're less likely to get hurt from overtraining or pushing yourself too hard. That's because you'll have greater self-awareness, and hopefully, more confidence.

The Ideal Coach

The ideal coach is a leader you can trust to guide you as either an athlete in an individual sport or a team sport.

According to a 1999 study from Michigan State University, researcher Deborah Feltz, PhD, and her colleagues determined that the best coaches, no matter the sport, effectively address four different aspects of competition: motivation, strategy, technique, and character building. Feltz and her colleagues then outlined the key strategies that pertain to each of the four aspects.

Motivation

A great coach will motivate you to bring out the best performance you are capable of as consistently possible. Dean Reinmuth, the teaching golf pro for professional golfer Ricky Barnes, and former teaching golf pro for Phil Mickelson, told me that he motivates his players by making sure the player has the proper skills and an honest assessment of his or her skill set before competing at a level or degree of difficulty of the course or a level of competition that is too advanced for his or her skill level. He told me, "Competing at a slightly higher level is good but attempting to play too far ahead of where one's skills are creates a feeling of defeat."

A great coach can also lessen a player's anxiety. According to researchers, a coach's positive approach during competition is not only motivating, it can lower athlete anxiety. What's more, a coach that has positive rapport with his or her players will feed the athlete's performance. A negative relationship—where a player feels bullied or tormented by his or her coach—can significantly contribute to a player's anxiety.

Feltz and her colleagues believe the following are integral for coaches to effectively motivate players:

- **Maintains confidence in athletes:** The confidence level of any athlete will be tested from practice to practice and game to game. A good coach will know how to teach athletes to adapt to various stressors in order to keep confidence at the highest it can be.
- **Mentally prepare athletes for competition:** A great coach knows how to assimilate the various resources athletes use (i.e. the roles he or she is taking on as outlined in this book) and gives positive feedback to show athletes that their hard work is paying off. A good coach will get the team to be at their physical and mental peak during the game.
- **Builds self-esteem:** The self-worth of an athlete is critical to their performance. A great coach will try to keep the negative self-talk at bay while building a sense of well-being.
- **Motivates athletes:** Understanding the drudgery of practice, a great coach will combat complacency by providing words of encouragement or changing up the routine.
- **Builds team cohesion:** A great coach will not only match the players' strengths so they complement each other, they will teach the players to act as one team, not individuals.
- **Builds self-confidence of athletes:** The ideal coach will create performance goals in order to increase an athlete's confidence.
- **Builds team confidence:** When a coach can create an atmosphere of trust within the team, then each player will be motivated to perform better.

Strategy

A good coach adjusts his or her demands to bring the best performance from each player. This is especially true in team sports, where coaches will quickly recognize when players are hot, and when they're not. Sometimes, players get frustrated with coaches in the heat of the moment, especially if the coach is taking you out of the game. However, it's important to listen to your coach, since you trust this person to make the right decision for the benefit of the team. There will always be times when we are not the best athlete in the field, and it is better for the team to allow another to do the task. Don't take it personally, but take it as a learning experience. Your turn will come.

Feltz and her colleagues believe the following are integral for coaches to create effective strategies for their players:

- **Recognize opposing teams' strengths during competition:** A great coach will pick up on what is working for the opposition and develop a strategy to get his or her athletes ready for it by either adopting the same strategy or determining how to defend against it.
- **Recognize opposing teams' weaknesses during competitions:** A great coach will teach athletes how to expose the weaknesses of their opponents and take advantage of them.
- **Understand competitive strategies:** A great coach will have more than one strategy to win and will be able to know when and how to use them.
- **Adapt strategy to meet situation of the game:** The ideal coach can readily make adjustments to the team's strategy if the team is losing. These are the contingency plans that have been developed and practiced to keep the team ready.
- **Make critical decisions during competitions:** Some coaches may get paralyzed by the pressure of the game: a good coach will be decisive no matter what the pressure.
- **Maximize each athlete's strengths during competition:** A good coach knows what each player brings to the game. He or she will put in players that expose their talents to benefit the team's overall performance. For example, there may be a player sitting on the bench that is better suited to defend the opponent than a starter.
- **Adjust strategy to fit the team's talent:** The ideal coach will be realistic as to what level the athletes can compete at. For example, if an athlete is participating in a Sector 3 sport like boxing on the Sports Grid, but is training at a Level 1 anaerobic exercise level, he or she

should not be expected to compete with an opponent whose work-outs are at Level 3 exercises since the strength levels are different.

Technique

A coach has to have some experience with your particular activity. Most great coaches were previously players. If not, they need to have a complete understanding of the fundamentals, along with a love and appreciation of the game. The coach is the one you turn to when you have questions about your performance. He or she will guide you through each practice and create a master plan that will get each athlete ready for game time.

Feltz and her colleagues believe the following are integral for coaches to improve each athlete's technique:

- **Demonstrates skills of the sport:** A great coach will be able to flawlessly provide instruction on the techniques and skills necessary for the sport.
- **Coaches individual athletes on techniques:** A great coach will not only look at the team dynamics for overall strategy but will work with the individual players on improving their technique for specific moves that will take them to the next level and will also benefit the team.
- **Develops athletes' abilities:** Through drills and scrimmages that replicate game time simulations, great coaches teach athletes the different scenarios they could encounter during competition, which enhances their abilities and gives them the best chance to compete at their highest level.
- **Recognizes talents in athletes:** The ideal coach will spot the potential for those athletes that have natural and/or learned ability in the sport at an early stage in their training. They will also be able to access the right roles on the team based on these talents.
- **Detects skill errors:** The coach will both find and correct flaws in the execution of skills.

- **Teaches the skill of the sport:** A great coach will focus on the fundamentals of the sport during practices to allow the athletes to improve the proficiency of the skills necessary to play. The coach helps develop your mechanics of the sport to perfection.

Character Building

Ethics in sport requires a strong moral character, which includes the virtues of fairness, integrity, responsibility, and respect. Fairness is the ability to make decisions that are not biased and are made in the spirit of the competition. Integrity means upholding the highest standard of ethics. Responsibility means being accountable for your actions on and off the field. Last, respect entails treating others as you would want others to treat you.

The best coaches continually comment that character building is the single most important aspect of coaching. John Wooden, Hall of Fame basketball coach for UCLA, once said, "Be more concerned with your character than your reputation, because your character is what you really are, while your reputation is merely what others think you are." Wooden created his famous "Pyramids of Success" philosophy, and was able to win 10 out of 12 NCAA championships, including seven in a row. He is best known for bringing out the best in his players on and off the court.

Feltz and her colleagues believe the following character-building strategies make for the best coaches:

- **Instill an attitude of good moral character:** With every interaction and teaching a great coach will inspire their athletes to do the right thing on and off the field.
- **Instill an attitude of fair play among athletes:** A great coach will only instruct their athletes to play by the rules of the game.
- **Promote good sportsmanship:** A great coach will inspire athletes to respect their opponent and be gracious, whether they win or lose.
- **Instill an attitude of respect for others:** A great coach creates a culture of winning and respectful teamwork.

Time-Out: Coaching a Team in Transition

One of my most memorable experiences in seeing what great coaching can do occurred when I was a Sports Medicine Fellow at San Diego State University. One of my duties was to cover the men's basketball team. At that time Steve Fisher was the head coach, taking on a team that had a terrible record, losing thirteen out of fourteen of the previous seasons. Coach Fisher knew what it took to win: he won the 1989 NCAA championship while coaching the University of Michigan. The transformation I saw during the year I was there was remarkable. Coach Fisher was able to earn the respect of the players, and made them excited to play for him. He attracted the top talent, made sure the players had the resources they needed, and ran impeccable practices. With each successive game, I could see the individual development of the players' skills, and more importantly, their character was building with Coach Fisher's guidance. I also witnessed real chemistry develop between the players. In the one year I was there the team's record improved to an impressive 21–12; the year before Coach Fisher arrived, the team had won just four games in the season.

The Secrets to Self-Coaching

If you take on the role of the coach, you will need to work on each of the four characteristics of great coaching: motivation, strategy, technique, and character building.

Motivation

One of my favorite sports quotes is from Michael Jordan: "I've missed more than 9,000 shots in my career. I've lost almost 300 games. 26 times,

I've been trusted to take the game winning shot and missed. I've failed over and over and over again in my life. And that is why I succeed."

One of the best ways to motivate yourself is to take the time to be reflective. That's what any coach really wants—it is for you to be aware of how you are feeling at any given moment. Typically, this can only be done after the game or competitive moment. It's a meditative moment, to really tap into yourself at a quiet time, and think about how you're doing, how you're performing.

A good coach is able to motivate during times of winning and losing. The best coaches appreciate the effort that went into each game whether the end result is a win or a loss. While the goal of winning is always there, the coach is typically more focused on the strides you are making toward that goal and how you are improving along the way. The truth is, it isn't about the result, it's about what is going to keep someone playing at their best level regardless of the outcome and, of course, to keep it realistic. As long as you do play your best in whatever it is, that motivation will come, and then it may open other doors for other things to achieve.

If you're taking the role on for yourself, reflect to see if you played your best, practiced your hardest, regardless of whether you won or lost. Sometimes you're just playing somebody, and even if you're having the best day ever, that person you're playing against might just be much better than you. As long as you bring your best performance, then that's great.

The way you will continue to motivate yourself will depend on whether you are participating in a team sport or a solo activity. There are two types of motivation: *intrinsic motivation* is the drive to do something for its own sake, while *extrinsic motivation* is doing something as a means to an end. Athletes involved in individual sports typically experience greater intrinsic motivation than their team-based counterparts, due to freedom to make decisions and their aptitude for autonomy. Understanding your motivations will give you the best chance for success.

A good coach can convince athletes to stay positive even when the odds are against them. When coaches focus solely on the scoreboard, players' anxiety increases, because players can't control the outcome on the scoreboard. Ultimately, anxiety undercuts self-confidence, which affects performance and takes the joy out of the game. Anxious athletes end up spending their energy worrying about losing instead of focusing on the competition, even though that single-minded focus is necessary for winning. The way to scoreboard success—and more importantly, to keep athletes encouraged and engaged—is to focus on what we can control, such as fundamental skills or following the game plan.

Mistakes result from taking chances, stretching limits, growing and learning. But coaches who overreact to mistakes cause their players stress and make them so nervous about their mistakes that they end up making even more. Or, players become so intent on avoiding mistakes that they play too tentatively.

You can motivate yourself during adverse times by learning how to control your effort and learn from your mistakes. Every single mistake is an opportunity. There may be a fundamental skill you forgot, or a play that you could have executed. Talk with your teammates after the game and you'll surely get some free insight. If you play an individual sport, see if you can have someone videotape your games, so that you can go over them later and see exactly what can be corrected.

To combat the effects of mistakes and reduce the fear of making mistakes, consider implementing a *mistake ritual*, a physical motion you use to remind yourself to get past a mistake and focus on the next play. The ritual may be as simple as brushing off your jersey to trigger the letting go process. It may be taking both of your hands and smacking your helmet. It can be any cue you can develop to get your mind back into the present moment to focus on getting ready for the next play. For example, in football, quarterbacks are taught to have "short-term memory": they must have the mental discipline to get over making a mistake as quickly as possible so they can make the next play without the baggage of thinking about the previous mistake.

Strategy

Whenever performance starts to go down, a good coach will shift gears and reassess by calling for a time-out and to regroup. By taking a break, you can change the momentum. We can do this ourselves in our sport, and for that matter, in any aspect of life. Call your own time-out when things are not going well. Reassess, consider changing to a different strategy, do a pep talk to yourself, do deep breathing, etc.

Let's say you're running a marathon and your hamstring starts to cramp. Step back a little bit. Even if you are going for a personal record, there will always be another chance. Instead, slow it down a little bit and regroup. When you start to feel better, then you can ramp back up again.

The ability to be self-reflective will affect your strategy to win. If you can be honest with yourself when trying to play your sport, without making excuses when you don't perform to the best of your ability, then you will be quick to accept your best efforts in any given moment. Regroup afterward and go over the situation to see if in fact that was your best effort. If it wasn't, then try to figure out what you can do differently next time.

Technique

Taking on the role of the coach will require some research: before you make further adjustments to your game strategy you'll have to learn everything there is to know about your chosen activity. Luckily, the sports world is rich in easily accessible resources. Beyond the books and the Internet, I've found that other players who are at a slightly higher level can provide the best insight into your game. Don't be afraid to ask questions from knowledgeable players. For example, I continue to improve my tennis game—even though I've been playing since I was four years old—by picking the brains of those above my level of play.

For example, when I was in the eighth grade I was brought up to the high school level to play tennis on the varsity team. I was flattered and scared about playing against the more experienced players. In an almost pestering way I constantly asked the rest of my teammates how to put more spin on the ball, how to stop myself from double faulting on key points, and how to hit a more consistent backhand stroke. The next year, our team made sectionals, and I was matched up against the number one player in the league who was being scouted to play college tennis. I kept remembering the fundamentals that I was taught and to tried to play naturally and freely, the way the older boys had taught me. Against the odds, I won that match, and I attribute the victory to the help of the much more knowledgeable players.

A second issue is overtraining. Overtraining is defined as an increase in the amount or intensity of physical activity combined with inadequate recovery time. While some level of overtraining is a prerequisite for peak performance, pushing yourself too hard can lead to fatigue and under-performance: when you are trying as hard as you can but not getting much better. This combination is often referred to as a state of physical *staleness*. Typically, those participating in individual sports become stale more often than team players. This could again be attributed to the individual athletes' greater autonomy, resulting in overambitious goals. When an athlete is overtraining, the longer they practice the longer it will take to recover, and without this balance you can find yourself with career-ending injuries. I see this in individual sports like triathlon competitions where an athlete has a difficult time ascertaining whether they are overtraining or putting in a subpar effort.

A good coach will be able to recognize when this occurs and provide the resources to allow for proper recovery. If you are coaching yourself, just having the awareness that overtraining can happen and can be a real cause of decreased performance will make you more accepting of that possibility. So if all of the other strategies and methods you are using are sound and being correctly executed, overtraining is the most likely cause of decreased performance.

In terms of technique, Dean Reinmuth suggests that athletes practice in front of a set of mirrors "where you can see your movements both face on and from the front and back." Another suggestion is Hudl (www.hudl.com), a free app with in-app purchases that allow you to watch slow motion videos of various sports professionals' technique and learn from them.

The Institute for Sport Coaching describes a great skill for making critical decisions. It's called the OODA Loop, which stands for Observe, Orient, Decide, and Act. *Observe* refers to the ability to single out meaningful data during a competition. There is so much to process during a game, athletes need to recognize what is important and leave behind what isn't. Then, the athlete is taught to *orient* the data, or assimilate the meaningful information into his or her next play. Once you have all of the information, then you can *decide* what the next steps should involve. Then, all that is left for the athlete to do is *act* quickly and with purpose. After the action, the athlete will loop back to observe again in order to assess the new situation.

Character Building

A good coach will not tolerate unethical play for the pursuit of the win. There is a difference between gamesmanship and sportsmanship. Gamesmanship means to win at all costs, even if it means actions that break the rules, or are simply unethical like faking a foul, for example. A good coach does not use gamesmanship as a means to winning. Sportsmanship is a more ethical approach. Aside from the competition, sportsmanship is seen as a means of cultivating personal honor, virtue, and character. It contributes to the respect and trust between competitors. The goal in sportsmanship is not simply to win, but to pursue victory with honor by giving one's best effort.

In order to build character, you need to work on the same four virtues of fairess, integrity, responsibility, and respect. To develop a sense of fairness, know the rules of the game, and play by them. Remember, there are no easy wins. To play with integrity means to engage in your sport in the context of the spirit of competition. Surround yourself with like-minded athletes that share your values. Read books written by coaches that show highly ethical behavior, such as John Wooden and legendary basketball coach Mike Krzyzewski. Take responsibility and be accountable for your actions: don't pass the blame or look for excuses. Lastly, show respect to your sport by honoring yourself, your teammates and your opponents.

Coaches Keep Athletes Focused and Track Their Progress

If you have a hard time keeping up with your goals or get easily distracted during practice, you need to ramp up your self-coaching skills. A coach not only keeps your eyes on the prize, but helps you stay focused and accountable. They are responsible for creating a schedule so that you can be sure to put in the time and energy to propel you toward success.

Time management is one of the best things a coach can teach an athlete. To my mind, the most impressive athletes are collegiate athletes. On top of having the responsibility to keep up with their schoolwork they have practices every day, travel games, and sometimes alumni obligations. They are able to manage this hectic schedule because they know how to make decisions that are based on what is most important at any particular moment.

To do this, go back and review your athletic mission statement and your goals. Once you're at the elite athlete level, your sport is supposed to take over your life. However, if you are not at that level, you need to keep your athletic activities in perspective. This means not losing sight of your overall life and other obligations, such as schoolwork, a job, or taking care of children. Creating balance is an important aspect of success. If you feel overwhelmed, which realistically can happen, take time to reassess your situation in the context of your sport and figure out how to prioritize what is important to you. Use your support system to help when necessary—nothing is ever accomplished alone.

There is no one perfect way to manage your time, but once you figure out a system that works for you, you'll find the time you need to achieve your goals. Some of my athletes rigorously keep their obligations clearly marked on calendars. Others create a reminder system using their smartphone or rely on the help of others. Building redundancies into your schedule is key in order to account for the inevitable unforeseen circumstances. For example, if tryouts for the baseball team you would like to make are coming up in three months, don't wait until two weeks prior to the start date to train. If you give yourself two months, you will have the proper time to ramp up slowly and safely.

A great coach will also collect data on each player in order to highlight areas of inconsistency or weakness. You can keep track of your progress as well. There are many metrics one can use to gauge progress, including monitoring gains or losses in speed, or tracking how well one plays against the same opponent over time (counting score, errors committed, etc.). You can create the right competitive environment to achieve your goals by setting realistic milestones. In Pat Riley's book, *The Winner Within*, professional basketball's legendary coach says, *"Excellence is the gradual result of always wanting to do better."* His goal for his players was not improving by 10 percent all at once. If he got a 1 percent improvement in five areas per player with a team consisting of twelve players, he would get 60 percent team improvement. In this way he believes, as I do, that every small step counts.

Clear attainable goals, like the ones we worked on in Chapter 1, are the key to success. For example, if you were a high school lacrosse player and now at thirty years old you have not exercised consistently, it is not reasonable to think you can go do a complete gym workout right off the bat just like you did during your high school days. Instead, start with a more reasonable goal of a ten-minute jog three times per week, increasing the duration by 10 percent per week, and slowly adding some of your old lacrosse drills.

Check in regularly with your mission statement and the goals we developed in Chapter 1. Then, after a training day, practice, or competition, do an objective and subjective measure of how you performed. Objective markers include whatever statistics are kept in your sport. For example, in soccer they would include: minutes played, goal attempts, goals scored. The subjective markers involve how you felt you played: did you feel like it was best performance, energy level, focus, etc. These subjective thoughts will remind you of the intangible side of sport so you can grow emotionally from it. Score your experience on a 1–5 scale.

If you are an individual athlete like a tennis player, objective measures include unforced errors, 1st serve percentage, double faults. Then track each practice game and then your competition. Subjectively rate yourself on how you feel you performed: was it your best? What was your energy level? Were you focused? Again, score your experience on a 1–5 scale. You can use this to rate yourself, and if you have a coach or hitting partner then you can also ask him or her to fill it out as well to get an outside perspective.

Lastly, set up celebrations for reaching your goals. For the majority of elite athletes the reward is mostly the heroic achievement, but to celebrate is also an important and often taken for granted aspect of goal setting. For example, if you need to work on your backstroke, set a time-related goal for showing improvement. Then, once you reach it, have a celebration, like going out for dinner, doing something special with friends, or taking in a movie. Then, set yourself a new goal, and a new reward, and start the process over again.

Use the following charts to record your efforts for one week. You can download this form from my website (www.stepupyourgame.nyc).

Objective Measures	Practice 1	Practice 2	Practice 3	Practice 4	Practice 5	Practice 6	Game
Measure 1							
Measure 2							
Measure 3							

Subjective Measures	Practice 1	Practice 2	Practice 3	Practice 4	Practice 5	Practice 6	Game
Performance	1 2 3 4 5	1 2 3 4 5	1 2 3 4 5	1 2 3 4 5	1 2 3 4 5	1 2 3 4 5	1 2 3 4 5
Energy level	1 2 3 4 5	1 2 3 4 5	1 2 3 4 5	1 2 3 4 5	1 2 3 4 5	1 2 3 4 5	1 2 3 4 5
Focus	1 2 3 4 5	1 2 3 4 5	1 2 3 4 5	1 2 3 4 5	1 2 3 4 5	1 2 3 4 5	1 2 3 4 5

Time-Out: Tracking Progress with Technology

It's easier than ever to act as your own coach because there are so many facets of training that can be automated, including online tools that act as progress trackers. One of my favorites is called Irunurun (app.irunurun.com). Irunurun is a simple, free, goal-setting tracker. You enter a goal, set the number of days per week you want to work toward it, and then report in each time you accomplish your task. At the end of the week it will tally up your progress. You can even invite your friends to set up a social aspect to hold yourself accountable.

Meet Olympic Coach Adam Krikorian

One of my all-time favorite team coaches is Adam Krikorian, head coach for the 2012 Women's USA Water Polo team, and the 2012 recipient of the Olympic Coach of the Year award. I first met Adam in 2009 after the team won the silver medal in the 2008 Summer Olympic Games. In 2011 I was traveling with the women's team to Shanghai for the World Championships, and we were heading into the competition as the favorites. Unfortunately, the players performed poorly, and we came in sixth place. At the last team dinner we tried to figure out why we lost. Adam asked one of the newer players what she thought was the problem. Boldly she said, "The team dynamic between the older crew and the new girls is not cool, Coach. It's like we're outsiders."

Over the next year Adam worked to bring the team together, practice after practice, tournament after tournament. He listened to the individual player's needs, making adjustments, keeping them motivated, and trained them just enough to keep them at peak performance. Most importantly, he masterfully had them achieve their peak performance at the right time and the right place: the 2012 Olympic Games where they won the gold.

I spoke to Adam at length and asked him what he enjoys most about coaching. He told me, "Before working with the women's team I was at UCLA as both men's and women's head coach for water polo. Now we're preparing for the 2016 games. I love working with young people to help them to reach their athletic dream while teaching them the important life lessons that go along with that. I also just truly enjoy working as a team to try to strive and reach a common goal. I don't think there is any greater feeling than reaching or achieving success and being able to share it with a group of people that you love and respect."

I asked Adam if he uses different coaching strategies with a team compared to individual players. He told me, "I don't think there's a difference necessarily. Even when I'm coaching a team sport, I coach individual players. But, I will say that when you're coaching a team sport athlete you have to encourage them to be socially aware of how their actions and their attitudes affect others and affect the entire group. That's honestly one of the biggest challenges of coaching a team sport. Obviously you want each individual athlete to reach their potential, but it can't be at the expense of the team. And that's one thing I always remind myself as a team sport coach. You always have the team's best interest in mind."

When I asked him who his coaching role model was, Adam said, "I wouldn't say there's one person that's really had the biggest impact on me, but I've drawn from so many coaches that have coached me, going back to my Little League coach, my swim coach, my football coach and my water polo coach. I've also drawn on some of the best practices of coaches in team sports and in individual sport all across the world, and through various sports. I've not only taken and learned from the things I like but I've also taken and learned from the things that I don't like. And that's helped to define my philosophy as a coach and as a teacher."

Adam's secret weapon seems to be working with videotapes of games. He told me, "Learning comes from watching someone demonstrate a skill set, indicating some of the actions. Then repeating those skills yourself over and over. Repetition goes a long way in mastering a skill. Watch as much video of the top players in your sport on the Internet."

Lastly, I asked him how integral he felt as a coach to an athlete's success. Coach Krikorian told me, "I would like to think I am integral, but I'm only a coach. You are only integral if the athlete believes that you are. That's an important element. The athlete has to believe that the coach is integral. Otherwise it is not going to work. It sounds simple but it's much more difficult to enact. The athlete has to know that the coach is there for a reason. That reason is to help them reach their full potential."

A Coach's Game Day Responsibilities

Coaches are responsible for helping their athletes during practice days as well as game days. During practices their goal is to mimic game situations by pushing an athlete to the point of perfect performance without going over the current limit an athlete has, thereby reducing the risk of injury, illness, overtraining, anxiety or depression. For example, if I was to self-coach and I wanted to achieve a five-mile run, and I've only gone to mile four in practice before, and I think that I can do the five, then I'm going to push myself to go to that level during the next practice.

On game day, the coach makes sure the logistical details have been addressed, the players are physically ready, and the equipment is present and accounted for. You can do the same by creating a portable checklist that lists your equipment, uniform, snacks, water, etc. Keep the checklist somewhere handy so that you can quickly make sure you have everything you need before you leave for your competition.

The coach's main role on game day is to inspire the athletes to play at their best. This typically starts with the pregame pep talk. This is a technique coaches use to make sure that every player is mentally ready to give it their all. When you're acting as your own coach, your pregame begins with a little self-talk. Read your athletic mission statement to remember why you are there to compete. Play some upbeat, inspirational music, or develop a small routine that you can do every time. For example, some athletes meditate, while others who are superstitious wear certain articles of clothing or jewelry. Whatever your ritual is, stick to it. Most of all, enjoy! When I'm ready to run a 5K, at the starting line, I go through the route of the race in my mind. Then I tell myself, "Remember to have fun. Remember the fundamentals. I've already done the research, and I've prepared myself for this moment. I'm ready to go."

During the postgame is really when the coach's expertise comes in. During the postgame, the coach recaps the events and relays how the players can use this knowledge in the future. Not immediately afterward, but in the coming days they can get under the proverbial microscope and work with the players so that they can make adjustments to do better next time. As a self-coach, this might include watching hours of film, or giving yourself more time for self-reflection. Spending a few minutes after each practice or game with your mission statement and goals fresh in your mind will allow you to "review the tape" with purpose. Analyze your play so that you can adjust according to your goals.

Hiring a Professional Coach

If you are not seeing progress in your game, and are not meeting your goals after following all of the instructions in this book for six months, you may want to start working with a professional coach. Do not delegate this role to a family member. While it's reasonable to coach your children playing recreational sports, there are many aspects of familial relationships that may prevent family members from unbiasedly providing you with guidance. It is better to keep your family as your cheerleaders or fans, and hire a real coach to train and take the lead for any potential athletic career.

The first thing you need to think about before you hire a coach is to determine exactly what your needs are. Don't go on a particular coach's reputation before you figure out what you need. If you need motivation, you might be better off with a sport psychologist. If you need technique, you might be able to work with a more experienced player. Review all of the other roles as well and see if your needs can be handled by a specialist, or if you really need a coach to be your manager. Then, during the interview process, make sure that they possess what professional coach Wayne Goldsmith refers to as "the six C's of coaching":

- **Clarity:** Can they express their vision clearly?
- **Composure:** Do they work well under pressure?
- **Confidence:** Do they inspire confidence in their players by "walking the walk"?
- **Credibility:** Do they have good results working with other athletes?
- **Character:** Are their personal values consistent with yours?
- **Communication:** Are they easy to talk to, and respond to your requests quickly?

Once they have met these requirements, hire or affiliate yourself with a coach who matches your temperament and personality. If you're a laid back guy, look for a coach who can provide a matching environment to the one you will thrive in most, and who can provide you with feedback in a way you will not only feel comfortable with, but will listen to. You should feel like you're not necessarily connecting with your best friend, but feel, "Wow, this person gets me and speaks my language."

There are many resources for finding the perfect coach. For example, if you're looking to get back into soccer and want to take some lessons, check out the local soccer leagues: there you'll find coaches that will offer soccer lessons or can recommend camps in your area. Swimming has a great network of coaches at local YMCAs. If you'd like to become a better fencer, the bigger metropolitan areas will have clubs that will welcome you to learn the sport they love. A great resource where you can find a coach for your sport is CoachUp. It is backed by 2015 NBA champion Curry. You can search, book, and even track your progress on www.coachup.com

Recognizing a Really Bad Coach

Having a relationship with a professional coach requires complete trust. You have to trust that their guidance will not compromise your health, your relationships with your teammates, or your values. You need to feel at all times that your coach knows what's best for you, and that their recommendations are legal and sanctioned. If you don't have that feeling, or if you're working with somebody who's noticeably dysfunctional, it's time to get yourself a new coach.

Unfortunately, the warning signs are not always clear. Watch out for any of the following with your team coach or one that you hire individually. These are all signs of unhealthy behavior that should not be tolerated:

- If there's blatant favoritism for certain players
- If their actions are dangerous

- If their actions are not in your best interest or the best interest of the team
- If there is any sort of hazing cloaked as a "ritual" or "rite of passage"
- If bullying, teasing, or ridicule is tolerated
- If their response to poor performance is taken to a personal level that is demeaning in public or in front of peers

CHAPTER 7
THE COMPETITOR

It's great to win, but it's also great fun just to be in the thick of any truly well and hard fought contest against opponents you respect, whatever the outcome.

—*Jack Nicklaus*

The word "compete" comes from the Latin "*com*" and "*petere*" which means *together and seeking*. The true definition of competition is in the spirit of this definition: a joint venture where your opponent is your partner, not the enemy. The elite athlete uses their competitors—whether they are individual athletes, members of their own team, or an opposing team—as sources of motivating energy necessary for achieving both their goals and their mission.

Competition gives meaning for taking the field. When we engage in any sport, we inherently try for our best performance. While the goal may be to win the game, the win is not necessarily the true goal of competition. If your mission statement is to play tennis to your highest potential, then your competitor is the resource you'll use to constantly challenge your notion of what your potential can be, so that you'll continually improve your level of play. And when a defeat happens, you'll have the tools for discovering ways to become better, based on the understanding of your competitor's skills.

However, most athletes—and their coaches—misunderstand the role of the competitor. Critics of competition point to problems such as escalating and unnecessary violence between athletes, and the promotion of poor character development brought on through a "winning at all costs" mentality. In both instances, these athletes are only focusing on the win, instead of understanding the full extent of the purpose of competition, which is to bring out the best in their own performance.

I view competition as the greatest way to develop a sense of fair play, positive character traits, and the skills that promote success on and off the field. The competitor is just as important a role as any other in the elite athlete's entourage for enhancing the quality of performance. The competitor provides a powerful learning tool that helps athletes view problems as opportunities. Most important, the right competitor makes competition more enjoyable and less stressful. If you can learn to view competition and your competitors in this light, it will motivate you to stay with your game longer and be inspired to improve.

The Qualities of a Strong Competitor

Tao philosophy states that a competitor is the adversary—or the adversity—that motivates you. Those athletes that subscribe this philosophy have a clear understanding that they "partner" with their competition in creating a rivalry that will test their limits. It raises their game to the highest level each time they compete. You learn from your competitor as you play against them, as they will learn from you.

Finding a competitor often occurs organically through an organized activity. If you play on a team, your coach selects your competitors. If you join a running club or a tennis club, they will match you with someone you can race against. For example, I can go anywhere in the country to play tennis and I can find a competitor based on my USTA rank. I know that I can enjoy playing against other 4.5 level players, and they would be happy to play against me.

If you are looking to add a good competitor to your entourage, look for someone who creates an atmosphere of harmony, even during the most intense matches. They do this by showing respect to their adversary through even the simplest gestures, like showing up on time for a match or a meet, and making a full commitment to take the game, race, or challenge seriously. A good competitor will also be a student of the game, who shares your passion, enthusiasm, and even your obsession for the nuances and strategy of the sport. This ideal competitor would also provide three types of motivation.

The Competitor as a Challenger

The ideal competitor provides a level of challenge that is moderately difficult, yet equal to your current capabilities. Competition is meant to bring out the best in your play, not provide an opportunity for a complete routing. If your rival plays at a level much higher than your own, the game will be frustrating. You can train with someone at a higher level so that you learn from them, pick up some skills from them, or be inspired by them, but to actually compete against them would be unsatisfying. And if you play against someone who doesn't have the same skill sets you do, you won't take the competition seriously. The reason why the Olympic Games are so compelling is because the best athletes in the world are challenging each other at the highest level. The evenness of the competition is what leads to breaking records, and some of the most memorable contests of all time.

Good competitors want to play against others who are at their best, because the better the competition, the greater the chance they have of experiencing a peak performance. For example, if your competitor has an issue with his or her ankles and can't really compete at one hundred percent, a true competitor would recommend postponing the match until the player was completely recovered: then and only then will the competitor perform on an even playing field to be able to determine who is best. Using the Sports Grid, look for a competitor who is in your same sector of aerobic and anaerobic capabilities. The most ideal competitor would be someone with whom you've shared this book, so that they are also working on their nutrition, their training exercises, their mental game, etc. That way you are both bringing the same philosophy to the competition.

Elite athletes get to know their competitors on and off the field. They study the training practices of their competitors, and analyze their games with other opponents. They discover what motivates their competitors, and try to determine what errors they make and how they can learn from them. They aren't necessarily copying their competitor's game, but applying this knowledge to their own style of play in order to remain one step ahead. Knowing your competitor's game plan gives you the advantage to devise a strategy to counteract any tactic they may use, as well as the chance to develop a strategy that your competition may not be adept at defending against. The truth is, what works for your competitor may or may not work for you—but knowing that information and testing it in your practice is important.

The Competitor Improves Your Game

A competitor is not only a rival; they can be your most valuable training partner. Without a real challenge, you will not gain the tools necessary to rise to the next level, or even gauge what the next level of play is. This holds true whether your competitor is someone on your team or someone from another team.

A good competitor on your team can motivate you, keep you accountable, and even push you harder than your coach or trainer. However, competition doesn't automatically enhance quality, especially if it is created in a pressure-filled environment. One common mistake athletes make when using a teammate as a competitor is that it can cause them to become shortsighted, relying on only a few good moves to get the win instead of improving all of the necessary skills for their game. For example, if a basketball player only goes to his best shot during practice, instead of developing and refining new ones, he might be able to perform well when playing against his teammates, but ultimately it will limit his overall skill development. A better strategy would be for the athlete to play against different competitors, even during practice, so that his skills can be tested through a number of scenarios. Invariably this type of training will lead to a stronger, more well-rounded athlete, not just a one-dimensional athlete.

The Competitor Enhances Character

Some athletes want to win so much that they lie, cheat, break team rules, and develop undesirable character traits that might enhance their ability to win in the short term but don't serve them well in the long term. These athletes are not ideal competitors, and frankly, it's not much fun to play against them.

Instead, it's much more compelling to play against a competitor with character. I believe that athletes who display a strong moral compass and play within the rules of good sportsmanship will perform better and more confidently, ultimately making them better competitors. The four virtues of character building that we used to assess a coach—fairness, integrity, responsibility, and respect—can apply to any athlete: you can show others that you have these skills by avoiding arguments with coaches, officials, and opponents, and respecting the opposing team or competitor's efforts. A good competitor maintains self-control at all times, and at the end of each competition, accepts the results graciously.

One of the most important characteristics of a good competitor is someone who makes the game fun. Even in the heat of the moment, most professional athletes understand that they are playing a game. This doesn't mean that you don't take yourself or your game seriously or that you aren't trying your hardest to win. Instead, a good competitor understands the context of their game. At the end of the game, a good competitor shakes hands and recognizes that their adversary is a friend, not an enemy. That's why in many sports, opposing teams can socialize together after a contest. Even on the professional level, competitors can be friendly. For example, when you watch the NBA players, they pick each other up off the court when they fall.

The late Vince Lombardi, the great coach of the Green Bay Packers and the Washington Redskins, once made a statement he would live to regret. His statement, "Winning isn't the most important thing; it's the only thing" has become one of the most memorable lines in sports. However, in his own memoir he wrote, *"I wish I'd never said that. I meant the effort. I sure didn't mean for people to crush human values and morality."* His point is that while winning is important, it's not the only thing. Playing with your best effort and character is the most important thing.

The Three Types of Competitors

Elite athletes know that there are three distinct ways to compete:

Competing Against Yourself

The ultimate goal of the sport experience is to challenge yourself and continually improve. Athletes who participate in individual sports, like running, swimming, or dance, are constantly refining their skills on their own. They are striving for their best time, their best form, or their personal record (also known as "the PR"). Even if you play on a team, you can compete against your PR as you try to attain your goals. For example, if your goal is to bench press 300 pounds, ten times, in order to make the line in football, that's what you will strive for.

Competing Against Idealized Standards

This type of competition is slightly different than competing against yourself. In this scenario, you are trying to reach specific benchmarks of superior performance in your sport, such as a four-minute mile, a 20-foot pole vault, a triple-double in basketball, or a 100-yard rushing game in football. Utilizing the roles of the entourage and studying how other athletes reached these idealized standards will give you the information you need to strategize your approach, as well as the best chances to reach your goals.

Competing Against Other Athletes

This form of competition is inherently focused more on winning than improving your game. In order to compete against others effectively, you need to establish a healthy rivalry that fosters a sense of excitement for your game. For individual athletes, this type of competition is what you have been practicing for. For team players, a rivalry forces everyone to play at their best. When the competition is tough, every player on the team can make a difference. The question is, are you going to be the one that steps up and takes control of the game and changes the momentum in your team's favor? Having a formidable competitor opens the opportunity for you to shine.

This type of competition can also occur within a team, where one athlete is competing against another for a spot or position. In a team setting, only a small percentage of the entire team earns starting positions. Of course, every athlete wants to be a starter, so competition per position requires you to perform at your best. If you are chosen as a starter you are the best at your position. If you are not chosen as a starter, your overall goal may change: now you have to work your hardest during practice to show that you are ready to compete at the highest level and add value to the team.

While you can use competitors to motivate you to step up your game, do not compare or evaluate your own progress to other athletes, especially those on your team. Comparing yourself to others does not give you a fair assessment of your performance because your progress is based upon your skill set. Comparisons can be inaccurate and worse, destructive. Performance comparisons can prematurely turn off otherwise talented athletes. For you to do your very best, you need to compete against yourself. Worrying about how another athlete is doing as compared to yourself can only interfere with your ability to reach your own goals. However, this is not the same as taking constructive criticism: you should always be open to learn new skills or techniques from your teammates who have already mastered them. This will help the entire team reach their goals.

Elite athletes try to remove themselves from locker room gossip. Don't put too much credence on what other athletes say about your play unless you trust that they have your best interests at heart. Instead, rely on your coach and your own self-assessment to judge your progress as well as your technique.

One of the most formidable competitors I have ever met, who seamlessly used all three types of competition at once, is super lightweight boxer Antonio Orozco, whom I met at his second professional fight in March 2009 when I was a doctor for the California State Athletic Commission. I was always intrigued by what passion some boxers possessed. Orozco was up against Juan Carlos Diaz, a formidable opponent. Antonio did his homework—he knew what style of boxer Juan was and had a great understanding of his game. Orozco beat him by a knockout.

After the fight I went to check on him and we got to talking about how he managed the win. He had an air about him that was confident but not cocky. Orozco said that while he had executed his plan, he did not take for granted his opponent and his game plan. He handed me a T-shirt that had his face and name on it; his corner man said to me, "Look out for this kid in the future."

For years I followed Orozco's boxing career. I noticed his trainers would provide him with a variety of sparring partners. He would compete against himself, always trying to do better than his personal record by setting the bar high trying to win each time by unanimous decision. He would compete against the idealized standard, which in boxing is easy—win by KO each time. And of course he used his internal competitive drive to compete against others, with the goal of winning each time.

The next time I met up with him I was covering his fight against Mike Perralta in June 2010. I was still impressed not only by his smarts but by his moves, anticipating his opponents' every gesture. He is now 23–0. He has had unanimous decisions or TKO or KO in all of his bouts. What's more, he continues to respect his competitors and elevate his level of boxing each time he goes out.

Using Competitors to Your Advantage

Can you name the top three competitors in your sport? The competitor is crucial to your entourage to ensure that you are consistently tested, so recognizing them is important to developing a multi-faceted approach to your game. The top competitors will challenge you by presenting their own strategies during each match, which will compel you to analyze your skills so you can adeptly react to their game. The top competitors will also keep your head in the game and prevent boredom. Even if you aren't ready to face them now, challenging them can be one of your goals.

Do you view yourself as a worthy competitor, either for players at your level or even for those top competitors? Visualizing yourself playing against the top competitors can provide you with confidence that radiates so that you are seen by others as a master of the game. Believing that you belong among the better players means that you have a chance of competing at the next level and can win. When you feel like you belong on the field, in the game, or on the track, it creates a new sense of excitement and enthusiasm. In this way you are using your competitors to increase your self-worth, which will naturally enhance your comfort during the game.

Meet America's Cup Winner Peter Holmberg

Peter Holmberg was born and raised in St. Thomas, US Virgin Islands. He first learned to sail at age four, and won the silver medal in the 1988 Olympics, which is the first—and still the only—Olympic medal ever won for the US Virgin Islands. He turned professional a year later, and since then has competed in three America's Cups, winning the 2007 event with team Alinghi from Switzerland.

The America's Cup is held roughly every four years, and is the oldest continuous competition in sport, dating back to 1851. Peter told me, "The great thing about the America's Cup is that it's a national challenge. It involves not just individual skill but also design. It's a technology and a human challenge. There's a very defined time, usually a three or four year period, which a team has to assemble all of the components."

Peter is one of the most intense competitors I've ever met. I first got to know him when he was with the Oracle BMW Racing team, competing for the 2003 America's Cup against the reigning champions, Team New Zealand. I was helping with the medical coverage for his team. Peter and I hit it off immediately since we are both from the Virgin Islands. As I got to know him I grew to respect his passion to compete at the highest level. For example, Peter desperately wanted to take home an Olympic victory to the US Virgin Islands. He hatched a plan to campaign for the 1988 Olympic Games in Pusan, South Korea. This campaign benefitted from his strategic planning, a longer fund-raising period and a two-year training regimen. Part of his strategy was to get to know the waters of South Korea. The year before the Games he competed in the Pre-Olympic Regatta. He finished eighth, and acquired a wealth of knowledge. His reconnaissance mission spurred two key decisions—to purchase a Korean-made Hyundai Finn, and to train in the waters of the Virgin Islands which best replicated the rough sailing conditions off South Korea. Holmberg's strategy worked. At age twenty-seven, Peter won the silver medal at the 1988 Olympic Games, the first—and only—Olympic medal won by the US Virgin Islands.

In 1992 Peter ventured into international match racing. He began as an unranked skipper, competing with wild card slots, but moved up the world ranks. By 1999 he was ranked No. 3 in the world. He reached the pinnacle of match racing—a No. 1 world ranking—when he won the 2001–2002 Swedish Match Tour Championship.

During the 2003 America's Cup I was on hand to prevent and treat injuries. His ability to keep his performance and the team's performance at its best was remarkable. He fully embraced the entourage strategy, and made sure to use all the resources the team had available as well as encourage his sailors to take advantage of them. Peter would encourage anyone on the team to utilize the medical clinic or work with our athletic trainer. If they needed osteopathic manipulative treatment, I would perform it on them before, during, and after competition. Peter would encourage the other sailors to work their hardest with the strength and conditioning coach. Because of his leadership, everyone around him was completely focused from the beginning of the race to the end of the each heat. Even during difficult times he consistently showed me how he would learn from each experience. That year, Oracle finished a close second in the Louis Vuitton Cup, the Challenger Series for the America's Cup. Even though the team did not win, Peter earned the respect of the winners, and was invited to join Team Alinghi for the 2007 campaign, which they won.

Peter is a master competitor because he would not only look at the tangibles of his rivals, such as competition tapes, scouting reports, and technology, but at the intangibles that were responsible for improving everyone's performance. For example, he was always monitoring how the different crews were interacting with each other. He told me that he would watch if the other teams were having fun or keeping the stress levels high. Peter would then gauge his own team's morale and bring in other resources. When there was team dissention an outside consultant was brought in to improve the way the crew treated each other.

I asked Peter how he was able to motivate his team. He told me, "The compelling drive of being in one of these teams is to work as a team. Each person wants to excel individually but also as a team, and win the ultimate competition. That's motivation itself and if you are a sportsman and you love to compete, that just happens.

"All the America's Cup teams have two squads so that we can train internally, and each member of the team is vying for a position. I'm not a fan of it personally. I think it's not as synergistic as another method of choosing your ultimate opponent or person but it does serve to motivate. I'd rather compete for the game, so no matter what I'll put my best foot forward and beat my opponent as best as I can. Rather than setting your goal to win the competition, set as your goal to do the very best you can regardless of the outcome. The beauty of that is, it takes away some of the pressure. I've found it to be one of the greatest techniques to reach your peak performance. I always set as my goal, my best possible results and achievements, and let that be my motivating force. Secondary to that is my goal, winning the competition to be on the podium as a winner.

"In the Alinghi America's Cup campaign in '07, it was not a perfectly scripted and explained selection process. It was more of a subjective decision being made. That became frustrating at times to play properly or to better my chances of winning it. That is where I just had to revert to keep my head on my shoulders and ponder about the whole scheme regardless of the outcome. I'm going to go out there every day and keep trying to get better and better in this great opportunity I've got. The bottom line that I understood, I think saved us as well, was to believe in team.

"I've competed individually, but when you're part of a team you've got to remind yourself that the ultimate goal is for the team to win. That also plays a part in how you mentally survive. That gets you through some of the hardships, the struggles along the way, and that's what kept me ultimately positive.

"Each person needs to find their own drive and style that helps them compete positively, and feel good about it, survive the ups and downs and continue to march on. I guess I have used both. I prefer the personal goals of achievement to be the best one, that's the most long-term, healthy, motivational forces that I've found. It's a wonderful way of pushing yourself through life.

"There are times where in the moments of glory you might say the ethics get overlooked. Ultimately in the end, as I step from team to team and hear how people's names or reputations are talked about, ethics is still deep in all sailors' priorities and beliefs. I'm proud to say that I think our sport does have high ethics. If you ask people to name the best sailors of all time, you're going to hear the most epic, fair guys names mentioned first. Not the guys that had the greatest story or the compelling victory that got into papers. I'm proud to say that sailing does have that as their core, and

I personally hold it very, very high. No victories are complete without a true, epic, fair play. No victory is complete without good ethics behind it."

I asked Peter to describe his ideal type of competition, and he told me he looks for a couple of qualifications. "First, a good competition has clear parameters with minimal boundaries to enter, and fairness is clearly established. Second would be a competition that combines both a physical and mental challenge. I think sport psychology is the one element still not fully appreciated in sport, mainly because of our machoism. It's the greatest element that I think is still untapped. I think it can certainly make or break a team, make or break a person. I see it consistently still being the number one element to success, in any sport."

Learning from the Best: The Army-Navy Football Rivalry

During my Family Medicine residency I was just getting my feet wet in Sports Medicine, and I went to Baltimore, Maryland to witness competition at the highest level: the annual classic Division I Army-Navy football game. The energy in the stands was simply fantastic, and I saw what the epitome of rivalries was like. This particular game is known as the best rivalry in all of college sports. It is not only one of the oldest football games, dating back to 1890, but it was also recognized as the ultimate showdown between some of the top collegiate athletes in the nation.

Afterward, I studied everything I could about how the athletes on both teams trained, how they practiced, and how they were motivated by the ultimate prize—to play their best football at this game. The training programs for both football teams are each connected to how they prepare to become the nation's military leaders. For example, back in 1944, Commander Thomas J. Hamilton, the head of the Navy's Preflight and Physical Training program and a former head football coach, thought football was the ideal way to train men for combat. Football then became an integral part of the Navy's overall training strategy, which continues to this day.

For many of the athletes this game is the culmination of their football careers. It represents their years of hard work, determination, and sacrifice. The discipline to not only incessantly practice, review tape, and team build is not all that matters—both Army and Navy players are required to maintain their academic responsibilities or they are not allowed to play. At the same time, they are training as soldiers or sailors every minute of every day year-round. They truly are America's best and brightest. The players all know they have the talent and ability, but the rivalry is what makes each game so compelling.

My favorite part of the game occurred at the end, when I witnessed one of the game's most honored traditions. First, the two teams join together to sing the losing team's alma mater. Then, both teams stand in front of the winning team's student body and serenade them with their alma mater. Everyone in the stands and on the field became part of the experience, and I felt that I was witnessing the best example of competition.

CHAPTER 8
THE ROLE MODEL/HERO

All the courage and competitiveness of Jackie Robinson affects me to this day. If I patterned my life after anyone it was him, not because he was the first black baseball player in the majors but because he was a hero.

—*Kareem Abdul Jabbar*

In November 2012 I was asked to speak about health to a few local youth water polo clubs who were training together just north of New York City. I was part of a panel discussion that included some of USA Water Polo Olympians from the 2012 London Games that was targeted to the players, ages eight to twelve, and their parents. My presentation was short and sweet and focused on being a team physician for elite athletes. Then the athletes each took the stage, and spoke about what it took to get to the Olympics: their determination, the tears, the long hours, and the triumphs and disappointments. The crowd was completely silent, even the children. Everyone was hanging onto every word as if these messages were the fuel that would energize them to make it to the Olympics themselves. Afterward, the kids got into the pool to do some drills with the Olympians, soaking up every ounce of not just technique and skill but inspiration.

At the end of the camp the athletes were asked to give out autographs and pose for photo opportunities with the kids. To my surprise, one of the younger boys brought over his water polo ball and asked me to add my name. I assumed he made a mistake, but the boy was determined to get my autograph, even though I insisted that I was not an Olympian. I looked at his father before taking my pen to the ball and said, "Really? Are you sure?" The father replied, "He wants your signature because you help them stay healthy." I felt humble to say the least, and then realized that this boy saw me as a role model.

Children spend a lot of time thinking about whom they aspire to be like when they grow up, and sports stars are often at the top of their list. Interestingly, many of the elite athletes I've come to know can also cite their own role models who continue to inspire them. For example, I've worked with some professional athletes who are currently playing against some of their own role models. For them this is literally a dream come true. In tennis Eugenie Bouchard, one of the top players in the world, had the opportunity to play superstar Maria Sharapova in 2014. In basketball, Dwayne Wade, NBA player for the Miami Heat, played his first game against one of his idols, Allen Iverson, known simply as "AI." After the game he admitted that he has been scared to play against his hero but also found it to be an honor. Wade used to practice the famous "AI crossover" as a teen.

When I was growing up, Björn Borg was my hero. I was very impressed with his five consecutive Wimbledon wins. He lived, ate, and breathed tennis, and that's what I wanted to do. I wanted to play like him, I wanted his poster, and his racquet, and made sure that I saw or read every interview he did. Borg was a shy guy and he didn't give many interviews, but whenever he did I would literally tell my family, "Everyone stop. I have to hear what he has to say" (this was back before DVRs). Each interview made an impression on me: I noticed that he was polite and kind, and always demonstrated good sportsmanship. He would habitually congratulate his opponent, win or lose. And if he lost, he was a graceful loser. I realized that his sportsmanship allowed him to show his best side even when faced with defeat. I looked up to that: when I lost, I became more gracious, and I noticed it helped me overcome defeat faster and get ready for the next match.

The impressions that I gleaned from following Björn Borg so intently have helped my tennis game in measurable ways, which is why I strongly feel that a hero or role model is an integral role in the elite athlete's entourage. I've found that remembering why one was inspired to follow in someone's footsteps can dramatically improve your game. In fact, I believe that the ability to stay connected with the role model we grew up with, or to be inspired by a new hero, is a key factor in achieving high performance.

Using Role Models to Your Advantage

I like to think of these heroes as an elite athlete's most secret weapon, because they are so underutilized. First, just thinking about your heroes makes you more passionate about your game, keeping you engaged in the game or your training program. We use their goals as milestones for ourselves, and those goals keep us moving forward. They also allow us to remember how much fun the sport is, as both a participant and a spectator. Remembering your hero's shining moment on the podium, their postgame interview, a funny moment on the field, or even their support for a charity to better the community—can keep you committed to your sport.

Heroes can also lend an air of companionship, which makes you feel less alone in whatever endeavor you're taking on. Knowing that someone else has taken on the same challenge and has reached a level of mastery you are searching for can provide the confidence you need to keep going. This person is already admired for pursuing the same accomplishments, and knowing this should propel you to continue to strive to reach your goals.

Strategically, you may become a better player as you emulate the techniques that your role model is best known for. In fact, you'll find that it's not just entertaining to watch them. You are going to improve your game because as you embody this person, you're going to figure out what made them successful. This could be their footwork, or their swing, their favorite equipment, or their character. As a teen, I used to wear the same headband as Björn Borg when I played tennis. I soaked up all his small idiosyncrasies, which added up to create a deeper level of engagement with tennis than many of the other athletes I played against.

Reclaim Your Hero

The ability to stay connected with the role model we had growing up or developed over one's life is a key factor in achieving high performance. One way to reconnect with the heroes of your youth is to talk with the people who were in your life during those time periods. For example, when I was so crazy about Björn Borg, there was a time that I wouldn't go to bed without my tennis racket. My parents still remember how obsessed I was. Hearing from them about how they interpreted my behavior allowed me to remember the feelings I had at that time.

It's also quite possible that over the years you've had more than one role model, especially if your athletic interests shift. You might even have had different role models for different aspects for your game. For example, I remember as a kid when John McEnroe used this unorthodox serve. All my friends tried to copy it. Today, if you want to play like Rodger Federer, you better work on your footwork. Stan Wawrinka, who just won the 2015 French Open, has a devastating one handed backhand, which is something that I've always aspired to achieve. He's my new role model for that skill, because I've always wanted to perfect a one handed backhand. It makes me want to strive to be better at my one handed backhand by watching his matches; I try to pick up the subtle cues of why his technique is flawless. I admire Novak Djokovic because he is tenacious. And I admire Maria Sharapova because she conducts herself with respect.

If you can't relate to your past heroes, choose new ones that have stellar records in their respective fields and who also strive to make a difference in their everyday lives. In a 2012 article entitled *The Greatest Sports Role Models over the Past 25 Years*, on CNN's sports website, bleacherreport.com, writer James Riggio included a little-known NBA player named Adonal Foyle on his list. Foyle had played college basketball for my alma mater,

Colgate University. His accomplishments on the court were impressive; however his life's work, founding Democracy Matters, a nonprofit, nonpartisan organization aims at spreading democracy throughout the world, was far more inspiring.

I speak with each of my patients about who their role models were when they grew up, and invariably the answer is often preceded by a long pause. I was once working with Seth, a patient in San Diego, who told me that besides his health issues he was having some financial difficulties. He was in trouble with his business partner and had turned to drinking as a way to cope. I met with the family and discovered Seth was also having marital issues due to his drinking. Seth was always active growing up, a cross-country runner and a swimmer in high school, had a decent upbringing, but he also had a family history of alcoholism. By starting him with the right outside interventions, we were able to get his life back on track.

Six months later Seth was still sober, and when he came in to see me we talked about his new goals. While he was working on himself, he realized how much he missed his athleticism. He also realized that it had provided a real grounding force for him growing up. We talked about how important running was to him and soon he wanted to get back into sports: Seth saw that having a new positive outlet would help him control his urges to drink.

Then I asked him who his idol was growing up. He recalled watching the IRONMAN Championships in Hawaii in 1985, and how the winner, Scott Tinley, had inspired him. Scott had completed the Nice Triathlon just three weeks before his win, and Seth remembered how inspired he was that Tinley was able to recover so quickly, train, and win the world's top IRONMAN prize. I asked Seth to watch that race again and come back to discuss it with me.

When he came back to my office, Seth told me he had felt that same sense of inspiration he experienced back in 1985, and wanted to give IRONMAN training a try. We discussed what it would take to be an

IRONMAN triathlete, and together we developed a plan to put the roles of an entourage in place for his training. He went on to try some sprint triathlons and soon got the bug.

I moved to New York shortly after seeing Seth for the last time. Now six years later, I ran into him when I was back in California for business. Seth told me, "Doc, I've been sober for six years now, my business is better than ever and my family life is solid with my wife and two kids. I have done two IRONMAN triathlons and have never felt better. Remembering that 1985 IRONMAN Championship was so important for me—it saved my life."

Time-Out: Getting Over the Disappointing Hero

Sometimes, our heroes disappoint us. You may even feel betrayed or misled. Sometimes, we have to recognize that the hero we fell for was not really representative of the whole person. While we'll probably never really know all of the complexities of our heroes, we do know that they are human, and as such, are bound to make mistakes.

Even though they have great moves, athletes who break the law, or the rules of their game, are not great choices for role models. You can aspire to play like certain people, but you don't have to aspire to be like them.

The Elite Athletes' Mutual Admiration Society

Most elite athletes choose a role model within their sport. However, I've come across a few athletes who have been inspired by other athletes outside of their sport. When the role model comes from a different sport or walk of life, it is usually the character, or mental toughness of that role model that the athlete finds compelling. For example, Usain Bolt has been a huge fan and supporter of NBA all-star Kevin Garnett. Bolt appreciates Garnett's level of commitment. He has been quoted as saying, "KG for me, he's a fighter, he's a leader, he's a champion. He's very tough mentally, and he goes out there and plays hard and always gives 150 percent. So for me, that's the biggest thing. Even when he was injured, he was always there with his team, always supporting them, always pushing them to be the best, so for me, that's something big. That's a leadership quality that I like and appreciate."

Becoming a Hero

The ultimate role is being a hero for others. Elite athletes understand that they are role models for others, and for many, just knowing this helps keep them on track of achieving their own goals. I've been told by many elite athletes that knowing there is someone idolizing them helps them maintain their skills. What's more, elite athletes do not take on the role of a hero lightly. On the field, they know that when others are watching, you have to play with passion and integrity. Off the court, most elite athletes understand that they are not solely defined by their prowess.

Knowing that you are a role model to someone else will also keep you on track to meet your goals. For example, if your goal is to be a faster runner, and you know that other people in your running club are looking up to you, you'll probably strive harder to reach your goal. It just adds more good fuel to your drive to continue that process.

You can also be role model for someone in your family, especially a spouse. According to a 2015 study conducted at Johns Hopkins University, spouses influence each other's exercise habits. When one spouse is following an exercise program, it significantly and positively influenced the other spouse to start exercising. If you have a spouse, family members, or friends who are engaged in a sport that you like, consider allowing yourself to be positively "peer pressured" to start. Ask them about what inspires them, what their training regimen is, how it impacts their life, etc. Their ability to be your role model can be your key to having fun and success in something totally new. Or, if you are actively engaged in a sport, see if you can get your spouse, friend, or family member to join in. You'd be surprised to find out that all they were waiting for was an invitation.

Meet Olympian Tony Azevedo

Tony Azevedo is a four-time All-American and NCAA Player of the Year at Stanford University, and has served as captain of the Men's Water Polo Team for the 2008, 2012, and is going for his fifth consecutive Olympics as team captain in the 2016 summer games. I first met Tony in 2010 when I traveled as the team physician with the men's USA Water Polo team for the World Cup in Oradea, Romania. I quickly realized he was a natural leader and knew what it took to perform at his highest potential.

Tony was born in Rio de Janeiro, and started playing water polo when he was eight years old. His father, Ricardo, was a member of the Brazilian National Water Polo team, and has led Tony as both a coach and a mentor. Ricardo coached Tony during his age group and high school career. Ricardo Azevedo was previously the US National Team coach, and is currently the coach of the Chinese National Team.

Tony told me, "The biggest thing for me growing up was my father. He was a big part of my life. He was probably my biggest role model. Even though our family had money in Brazil, he moved us to the US with the dream of being an Olympic coach and doing something big in the United States.

"I played baseball growing up. My father liked sports, and he really loved baseball. But I also went to my dad's water polo practices, starting when I was eight, nine years old, just getting in the water and playing with the team. It wasn't until I was fourteen at the '96 Olympics when I went as a ball boy that I was struck by the power of water polo. I remember sitting there and watching the games. I specifically remember being on the bench behind the Spanish team right before they won their gold medal. Just seeing the fans and seeing what it meant to those guys and the emotion that they were going through stuck with me. Even today I talk about that story and I get goose bumps. I knew at that moment that all I wanted to do was to represent my country in the Olympic Games and that I wanted to win a gold medal. I wanted to feel what those guys felt. Right then, I decided, that I'm going to do whatever it takes to be an Olympian. Four years later, waking up every morning at 5:00 a.m., drastically changing my body and increasing my speed and skills, I made my first Olympic Games.

"The journey has been wonderful. Luckily I had a great career after graduating from Stanford. After my second Olympics I moved to Europe, where I played for ten years. Now I'm playing in Brazil and every Olympic team has been different. Hopefully, I can end this career with a gold medal in Rio.

"My dad really helped guide my life. I knew he always had his head on straight and always talked to me about how important education is, how important working as hard as you can is. I saw it firsthand when we moved from Brazil and he was working three or four jobs just to support our family. I saw what it meant to him and I knew if you want to be successful at anything, you have to work at it.

"I was there on the bench behind the great player Manuel Estiarte when he won his gold medal. He is the only six time Olympic water polo player in history. He was a small guy and I knew I was never going to be a big, big strong guy like these other guys. Manuel was smart, fast, and he was the team's leader.

"I also want to be successful in my career as well as being a good father, just like my father was. I was lucky enough to have two role models that really were positive influences in my life. Every day during training I would think about either my dad as a coach or Manuel Estiarte as a player, both of whom worked so hard. They never got tired, and I thought, *I can do that*. I definitely think that if I didn't have such great role models I don't think I would be the same person I am today. They formed who I am and kept me going in the right direction toward my ultimate goal.

"I also realize that I am a role model. People don't realize that being a successful athlete, there comes a lot more than just getting out on the field and playing hard. The fans and the kids look up to you, and I know that if my actions were negative, it would upset them. When I was younger, even in college, I didn't really look at myself as a role model because I was still shaping myself, and finding who I was, and trying to accomplish so many things. I remember going to the 2004 Olympics, and Manuel Estiarte was already trying to be a part of the International Olympic Committee. I was walking into the dining hall, and I remember him pulling me aside to introduce me to someone and saying, 'This is the next Manuel Estiarte, the next big player in the world.' I won't forget that. It was one of those things where I was like, *Wow. This guy actually thinks I could do something like him to help change the sport.* To me, that was one of the most gratifying things I ever heard.

"After we won the silver medal in 2008 I started doing clinics and camps and reaching out to kids. I've seen how I've influenced them, and some of the kids even write to me, telling me how something I said changed their life. I can remember traveling somewhere once and a mother came up to me and said, 'Look, you told my son years ago to never give up, and how important education was, how to set goals. To this day he's taken that to heart. He went home. He wrote those goals on a piece of paper. He's accomplished everything, and he just got into the school of his dreams. I want to say that you made that difference in his life.' It's an amazing feeling. I realized that just like I had great role models, I am one of them now. I know that I'm going to be a role model for my son. It comes full circle.

"Being a role model makes me think twice before doing some things. Also, I try to reach as many people as I can. I had a great role model and I think the more kids I can inspire, the more kids I'm the role model of, the better for them. The better for our sport."

CHAPTER 9
THE PSYCHOLOGIST

The ideal attitude is to be physically loose and mentally tight.

—Arthur Ashe

The elite athlete uses their mind as yet another tool in their arsenal that can help enhance their performance. Their mental game is just as important as their physical one, and they recognize that their mindset requires specific training. This is why a sport psychologist should become an integral part of every elite athlete's entourage.

Burton Giges, MD, past president of the Association of Applied Sport Psychology and clinical professor in the Athletic Counseling Program, Department of Psychology at Springfield College, Massachusetts, found that athletes succeed when they can focus on developing their potential in the long run, and at the same time are able to attend to what he calls "here-and-now experiences" of competition. Athletes also need to be comfortable with risk-taking behavior, while at the same time take responsibility for their choices.

Giges believes that all athletes have the inherent capacity for optimal functioning, and would be able to do so if nothing stood in their way. His focus, which I agree with, is to remove the psychological barriers athletes often develop in order to release their potential. He refers to this technique as "clearing the way." These barriers happen to all athletes at some point in their career, and don't necessarily mean something is wrong. Barriers don't always require help from others to remove or get through, and while they may not be obvious, they are important to remove.

According to Giges, there are four types of psychological barriers:

- **Cognitive:** (thoughts, beliefs, opinions, judgments, expectations, attitudes): self-doubt, self-criticism, low self-confidence, low self-esteem, perfectionism, blaming
- **Affective:** (emotions, feelings): anxiety, guilt, sadness, anger, shame, embarrassment, disappointment, emotional hurt
- **Behavioral:** (action or inaction): overtraining, impulsiveness, giving up, pushing too hard, getting into fights, poor communicating
- **Conative:** (pertaining to issues of striving or desire): conflicting wants (personal vs. others, sport vs. other interests), low motivation, excessive desire

Giges describes some of the most common psychological barriers seen in sport performance: anxiety, low self-confidence, anger, self-criticism, low self-esteem, shame, loss of incentive, and difficulty staying focused. The process of removing these psychological barriers involves identifying them, exploring their meaning, and initiating a change that will decrease their impact. For example, in golf, a common performance anxiety can lead to the "yips," an involuntary wrist spasm that occurs when putting. When players try to hit a really easy putt that they keep missing, they inadvertently place a load of psychological barriers on themselves that keeps them from performing at their best. Instead, they're stuck in this mode of thinking, *Oh no, I'm now not performing well. Oh no, what are people going to think? Oh no, what's my ranking going to plunge to?* One of the most famous examples happened with Phil Mickelson when he was on the eighteenth tee at the US Open at the Winged Foot Golf Club. He had the lead going into Sunday, but ended up shooting a double bogey on eighteen when all he needed was par to win; that year Geoff Ogilvy was crowned champion.

The yips aren't reserved to golf. New York Yankees second baseman Chuck Knoblauch was a Rookie of the Year, won several World Series rings and went to four All-Star games. But after all those achievements,

Knoblauch started having problems throwing the ball to first base, a routine and relatively simple task for any second baseman. In 1999 he had a total of twenty-six errors. Like other cases of the yips, there was no outward explanation for Knoblauch's loss of throwing ability.

Sport psychologists address both individual and team dynamics. One of the first sport psychologists I worked with was Peter Haberl. His current title at the USOC is senior sport psychologist in charge of team sports, but Peter was also a professional hockey player in Austria for nine years. At the USOC, Peter's role is to make sure that USA Olympic teams have the best psychological support so that each athlete can perform at their highest level.

Peter and I once traveled with the USA Water Polo men's team to Oradea, Romania, for the World Cup. Our team had just lost a crucial game during a preliminary round and morale was palpably down. The coaches knew if they did not reach at least fourth place their USOC funding might be in jeopardy. Both the players and the coaches recognized that they could, and should be performing better: most of the men were part of the same team that brought home a silver medal at the 2008 Beijing Summer Games. As a result, Peter was called in to meet with the players.

For the rest of the tournament, along with the practices and training sessions the coach and the athletic trainers set up, Peter would meet with the team as well as have individual sessions with team members. The players would also ask for "time with Haberl." After a week or so, team morale seemed to go up, and even the athletes who seemed to have the most issues were performing better at game time.

At the end of the tournament the team was scheduled to play against Romania, the host country, where the sport is as popular as football is in the US. The game was going to be shown on national TV, the stands were filled with Romanian flags, and television newscasters were everywhere. It also happened to be the game that we needed to win in order to be guaranteed fourth place. The game was close in the beginning, seesawing back and forth. But in the third quarter we started to score more frequently, despite the Romanians' increase in intensity. Even when the injuries started to pile up the coaches and players seemed to possess a unique sense of calm. The team stayed focused to the end and pulled off a much-needed win. The role Peter played in having the team gain the mental edge was apparent to me—he played a vital role in the win.

The Sport Psychologists' Best Practices

There are various approaches Burt Giges, Peter Haberl, and other elite sport psychologists use when they are working with teams or individual athletes to create better outcomes for competitive readiness. Regardless of whether you have relationship or unresolved personal issues that keep you from performing at your best, following the protocols a team psychologist provides will help you feel less alone or disconnected as you pursue your goals. They are an integral role for any athlete's entourage, because they will help you keep from becoming distracted by life's stresses that keep you from performing at your best. In order to really succeed, athletes have to know the triggers that can take them out of their game, and have the tools ready to quickly get back on track when these triggers occur.

The following methods may improve your game as you learn to change your mindset. Once you understand how each of these tools work, you can then choose from them when you are faced with a particular circumstance where calming anxiety or reducing negative self-talk is critical for success.

Mindfulness

One of the most effective tools a sport psychologist will teach is the practice of mindfulness: clearing our thoughts of everything besides the present moment. Your behavior or performance is based on the physical bridge between our inner experience and the outer world, and between ourselves and others. Mindfulness is an important skill to add to your arsenal so that you can concentrate on the present—your behavior on the field—instead of ruminating about the past.

Mindfulness practice involves learning how to simply and nonjudgmentally observe your own breath, body or thoughts. By emphasizing a focus on the here and now, mindfulness can train you to stay on task and avoid distraction. A mindfulness practice can change the structure of the brain so that you can pay attention better, improve memory, decrease stress, and increase overall happiness. Peter Malinowski, PhD, a psychologist and neuroscientist at Liverpool John Moores University, in England, was quoted in a recent *New York Times* article: "For some people who begin mindfulness training, it's the first time in their life where they realize that a thought or emotion is not their only reality, that they have the ability to stay focused on something else, for instance their breathing, and let that emotion or thought just pass by."

Sport psychologist Michael Gervais has trained elite athletes including the Seattle Seahawks and USA Beach Volleyball's triple gold medalists Kerri Walsh-Jennings and Misty May-Treanor. He uses mindfulness to cultivate confidence in what he describes as "full presence and conviction in the moment." When athletes can perform with confidence, they are more resilient when faced with setbacks, and can perform with an open mindset that allows them to see many more options available during each play.

According to Richard Carmona, MD, author of *Canyon Ranch: 30 Days to a Better Brain*, the signature trait of mindfulness training is to increase your capacity to observe everything within and around you. By doing so, it keeps you from being mindlessly swept away by emotions, worries, or preoccupations. It also helps to keep you from snapping to conclusions or making judgments. A mindfulness practice also allows you to notice the judgments or psychological barriers you habitually make, and by recognizing them, you can begin to free yourself from those judgments. Carmona says, "If you tend to be hard on yourself, mindfulness is a wonderful way of learning to be kinder to yourself. If you tend to be overly critical of other people, mindfulness can also help you to notice those judgments and develop a better attitude of kindheartedness."

A formal practice consists of structured experiences like meditation. Psychologist Amishi Jha, director of the University of Miami's Contemplative Neuroscience, Mindfulness Research and Practice Initiative, trains United States Marines to use mindfulness to achieve greater mental resilience. In the same *New York Times* article Jha was quoted as saying, "We found that getting as little as twelve minutes of meditation practice a day helped Marines keep their attention and working memory—that is, the added ability to pay attention over time—stable. If they practiced less than twelve minutes or not at all, they degraded in their functioning."

Many of the meditations in this book can be considered mindfulness meditations, especially the ones that have you focus on your breath. The following exercise was provided by the UCLA Mindful Awareness Research Center. Their website (www.marc.ucla.edu) offers a set of free guided mindfulness meditations. Have someone read you this meditation with your eyes closed. Or, you can record the meditation and play it back to you.

Close your eyes. Begin this meditation by noticing your posture. You may be standing, or sitting, or lying down. Notice your body, exactly as it is, and see if you can tune into any sensations that are present to you in your body in this moment. There might be heaviness, or lightness, pressure, weight. There might be vibration, pulsating, movement, warmth, coolness. These sensations can be anywhere in your body, and all you have to do is notice them. Notice what is happening with curiosity and interest.

Take a breath. As you breathe, relax. Not much to do except to be fully present and aware. Now let go of the body's sensations and turn your attention to the sounds inside or outside the room. There may be all sorts of sounds happening: loud sounds, quiet sounds. You can also notice the silence between the sounds. That the sounds are coming and going. Notice them coming and going. One tendency of our mind is to want to think about the sounds, to start to make up a story about the sound, and then have a reaction to it, "I like it, I don't like it." See if instead you can simply listen to the sound. Notice it with curiosity and interest. The sounds are coming and going.

Focused Attention

Focused attention is the ability to stay concentrated on a single topic or task, and when your mind wanders, bring it back as quickly as possible. This is different than mindfulness, where you become aware of everything that is around you. It is an important skill for any athlete to have because the more focused we are, the more successful we can be. Poor focus leads to unrest and self-doubt. When you are ineffective, you may feel guilty and frustrated with your lack of ability to stay on task, which then shakes your confidence overall. Yet when we improve our self-esteem, we achieve better focus.

The most efficient people don't really multitask. They are able to do one task, be fully present for that task, then move on to the next task, and stay focused on that task, without the baggage of thinking about the previous task. Focused attention teaches you how to manage disparate tasks and in quick succession. The ability to put one hundred percent of yourself into a single moment is the goal. Switching from one task to the next without hesitation and with ease allows you to get into a groove. When you are efficient, you'll feel more confident and start to develop a belief that you can accomplish the tasks placed in front of you, and do them well.

We can enhance our ability to focus just like we can enhance our muscles. The more we work on it, the stronger it becomes. I find that the athletes who are able to stay on task without getting distracted are less likely to succumb to negative self-talk and performance anxiety. For example, if a basketball player has trouble at the free throw line, the focus attention exercise would train the player to stay relaxed when it's time to take the shot, focus on the target, and to trust his or her arm without thinking how the basket would affect the outcome of the game.

I practice focused attention when I'm faced with a stressful situation, like a test, even if it's only a test of patience. My technique is that I "gamify" difficult situations so that it feels like I'm playing a game instead of pulling myself down because of the drudgery of the stressful situation. Psychological barriers in the form of negative self-talk will thwart my success. Instead of getting worked up and thinking my life depends of the outcome, I focus my attention on the task at hand and tell myself, *This is a game*. With this mindset I can reconnect with the child inside of me, and instead of getting anxious I become excited, and know that, "Hey, I really, really, really want to do well," as opposed to saying, "Oh, my God, if I don't do it well, then I'm not going to feed my children." I use that to my advantage, to be mindful and stay present with my inner child.

Practice the following focused attention exercise each day, or even during a time-out:

Sit in a comfortable centered position and focus your attention on just one thing. This focal point could be your breath, a mantra, or an image. Pay attention to what's coming in through your five senses (what you're seeing, hearing, tasting, touching, and smelling); how your body is feeling (heaviness, lightness, tension); to your thoughts, and to your emotions.

When your mind wanders away from the focal point, notice your new thoughts with an attitude of openhearted acceptance, and then come back to your focus again. You can acknowledge the extraneous thoughts, but then let them go so that you can return to your focal point. Instead of pursuing these lines of thought, just notice that you had the thought by saying to yourself, "I just had a thought." And then, gently let it go and come back to your focal point. The idea is to not engage in the new thoughts and instead become aware of the process of awareness itself.

Learning to Play Unconsciously

According to Vikram S. Chib, an assistant professor of biomedical engineering at Johns Hopkins University, how someone frames a high-pressure situation, and whether winning or losing is emphasized, can affect performance. Competition is not about winning. Rather, it is a showcase for each athlete to do their best. Every athlete has self-defeating, anxious feelings when they play, especially if you believe that you are in the heat of a battle. Being aware that these feelings will occur and accepting it as part of the experience is the key to being able to relinquish their control and instead convert that energy into a positive tool. The best athletes can do this and feel like they are in a state of peace, or playing "unconsciously."

The best athletes are said to be playing "unconsciously," meaning that they are playing effortlessly and not overthinking their strategies. They can do this because they're not letting their insecurities affect their performance. By slowing down and deliberately lowering your breathing into your diaphragm, you can train yourself to calm down when you're getting nervous. This kind of regular practice will enable you to calm yourself down quickly.

Try the following exercise:

Inhale slowly through your nose to a slow, comfortable count of four, filling your lower belly with the air. Hold your breath to a comfortable count of four. Then slowly exhale through your mouth to a comfortable count of six. Repeat this sequence, being sure that you remain comfortable throughout, without getting light-headed. If you find yourself getting dizzy then adjust your count both on the inhale and exhale until you feel more comfortable.

Maximizing Short-Term Memory

When you play with "short-term" memory you can separate mistakes from the past so that you can refocus on your current and future performance. One of the best ways to do this on the field or during competition is to take a time-out. Creating the space for transitioning away from the negative experience or memory is key to moving on. The problem for most athletes, though, is that even when time-outs are called, they may have difficulty actually taking the time to regroup.

Eckhart Tolle, a leader in self-help/spirituality and author of *The Power of Now*, describes short-term memory perfectly. One day he was at a pond and saw two swans swimming in harmony. All of a sudden, the swans got tangled up and appeared to be fighting, wings flying around with their bills darting at each other like spears. A few minutes later they swam apart for a moment, then started swimming together in harmony again, as if the altercation never happened.

In Chapter 6, we discussed creating a mistake ritual as a technique for quickly moving past a bad play or a loss. This is another way to create a short-term memory outlook during a competition. Once the mistake ritual is completed, you'll be better able to move forward during your game, leaving the problem to be analyzed later.

You can improve your short-term memory and utilize time-outs more effectively by following this quick protocol, which puts together all of the above lessons, instead of just standing around, catching your breath:

1. Focus on your breath.
2. Recite your athletic mission statement in your head.
3. Listen to your coach with focused attention. If you are playing an individual sport, self-coach and review your game plan and your options.
4. Let go of negative thoughts by using your mistake ritual.

The 7/10 Rule

When you are in a high pressure situation, like making a potentially game-winning play or racing to the finish line, it's important to have an internal barometer to measure your current stress levels, and to recognize the fact that when a particularly high level is reached, performance will surely suffer. I started using a scaled approach for my patients with anxiety, and have found that the same scale can help athletes maximize their performance.

On a scale from 1 to 10, if zero represents no anxiety, and 10 is a panic attack, developing a sense of what 7/10 feels like is crucial. Once you go over 7/10, the likelihood of having the wherewithal to use the tools you have developed is low. Make sure to be aware of your anxiety and if you become conscious of the fact that you are approaching a 5 or 6/10 on your anxiety meter, use any of the tools to bring your anxiety to a 1–2/10.

Music as Performance Tool

Another way I've been able to help my athletes focus is by utilizing music. Studies have shown that listening to music during exercise can improve results. Researchers have also found that some music is simply better to listen to than others, especially when it comes to creating a cardiovascular workout. For example, Dr. Costas Karageorghis, PhD, an associate professor of sport psychology at Brunel University in England, found that the most important elements in choosing the right music to accompany exercise is its tempo: the sweet spot is between 120 and 140 beats-per-minute which interestingly corresponds to the average person's heart rate during an energetic workout. FIT Radio has taken this one step further: it's an app that provides music based upon the kind of workout you want and the genre of music that appeals to you.

Listening to the right music can increase your pregame focus, and will certainly inspire you to do your best. In 2015, Canadian researchers found that when athletes played their favorite music during training, their exertion levels reduced and their commitment to their program increased, when compared to listening to no music at all. The study also found that regardless of your musical taste, listening to your choice of music could improve your enjoyment of your sport as well as improving performance.

It's no surprise that so many elite athletes have a pregame ritual that includes music when they're getting ready for the game. Both Michael Phelps and LeBron James would enter their respective stadiums with big headphones. According to Karageorghis, when athletes are very closely matched in ability, music has the potential to elicit a small but significant effect on performance. His research has shown five key ways in which music can influence preparation and competitive performances:

- **Dissociation:** Music can narrow attention, diverting the mind from sensations of fatigue, which in turn lowers perceptions of effort and promotes a more positive mood state. When this occurs, vigor and happiness become heightened, while negative aspects such as tension, depression, and anger are diminished. The physical effects of music are more prominent during low and moderate exercise intensities. During a more physically taxing session, music has limited power to influence what the athlete feels, but it does have considerable leverage on how the athlete feels.

- **Arousal Regulation:** Music alters emotional and physiological stimulation and can be used prior to competition or training as either a stimulant or a sedative, fostering an optimal mindset. Most athletes use loud, upbeat music to "psych up," but softer selections can help to "psych down," as well.

- **Synchronization:** Research has consistently shown that the synchronization of music with repetitive exercise is associated with increased levels of output. This applies to activities like rowing, cycling, cross-country skiing, and running. Musical tempo can regulate movement and prolong performance. Synchronizing movements with music also enables athletes to perform more efficiently, again resulting in greater endurance. The implication is that music provides temporal cues that have the potential to make athletes' energy use more efficient.

- **Acquisition of Motor Skills:** Music replicates forms of bodily rhythm and many aspects of human locomotion.

- **Attainment of Flow:** Self-selected music and imagery can enhance athletic performance by triggering emotions and cognitions associated with *flow*, defined by positive psychologist Mihály Csíkszentmihályi as, "Being completely involved in an activity for its own sake. The ego falls away. Time flies. Every action, movement, and thought follows inevitably from the previous one, like playing jazz. Your whole being is involved, and you're using your skills to the utmost."

Meet Sport Psychologist Burt Giges

When I interviewed Dr. Burt Giges, I asked him to share his specific technique for clearing psychological barriers. He shared the following that I believe every athlete can incorporate:

"The beginning of change can be very subtle. Most people think of change as behavioral change, but when it comes to psychology of change, often the key beginning is awareness. If I can initiate a change by helping them become more aware, that counts for me. I look for that in every session, with every client, with every athlete. I understand, and I identify what's in the way, and can I help them initiate a beginning.

"Then, I pay very close attention to language. I believe that language not only expresses what an athlete is thinking, or feeling, or wanting; it also contributes to it. For example, any athlete, when they know how to do something, and they screw up, they'll say, 'I'm so stupid.' They're expressing their disappointment, their frustration, dismay. They don't realize they are also contributing to the problem, because they are diminishing their self-esteem and their self-worth, and that will affect their motivation and their effectiveness.

"Sometimes a single critical question can help shift the person's perspective, initiate a change, which can be very meaningful. For example, I once treated a badminton player who realized that while he was an elite, competitive, successful athlete, he was more interested in going to medical school than in continuing in sport. But he was afraid that he would disappoint his parents, because they had put so much time, energy, and money into getting him training and matches all over the country. I asked him a question. It's a kind of question that can be a turn around. 'You think your parents would be disappointed, if they knew you are interested in medical school?' And he said, 'Oh, no. They'd love it.' I said, 'Okay, so what you can do is, instead of thinking of it as leaving badminton and disappointing them, you can now think of giving them even greater satisfaction and pride with your attendance of med school.'"

When I asked Giges what he felt about guided imagery, he shared the following: "I see mindfulness awareness as non-judgmental observation, which is an early step in a sequence that can lead to performance enhancement. Once I was working with an elite miler, who began to drop out at the end of her races, even though she might have been among the leaders.

"I had her close her eyes and mindfully visualize her last race, where she, in fact, dropped out in the home stretch because someone passed her. As she's telling me this, I interrupted her, and I said, 'What just happened?' And she's narrating dropping out. She said, 'I felt terrible shame.' Shame, as you might know, is a pretty early and deep-seated emotion. I asked, 'Was shame a familiar experience for you?' Immediately, she said, 'Oh yes.' She went right back to age six. Mind you, I didn't ask her how old she was. As a soccer player, she was the best and fastest soccer player on her six-year-old team. She gets the ball, and she's running down the field with the ball, and she trips and falls. Her father, from the sidelines, says, 'You stupid idiot! You could have made a goal.' She's overcome by shame. That's a single trauma, which is not usually an explanation. Usually, it's a representation of repeated experiences. It's a key memory, but it's not the whole explanation.

"Then I said, 'I want you to go through the shame race again slowly.' So she starts the narrative again. She gets to the point where the other runner, is passing her. The other girl beats her to the finish line. She finishes. She opens her eyes and says, 'You know, that didn't really happen.' I said, 'Yeah, I know.' She says, 'Well, what did happen? How come the second time I did it, it was different from the first?' I said, 'I'm not sure, but sometimes, when you bring something to the surface that was buried, it loses its impact. It loses its grip on you, even though you still remember it.' She never again dropped out of a race."

Sport Psychologists Address Real Mental Health Concerns

There are specific instances athletes face that cannot be self-corrected, and a professional psychologist needs to be engaged. These can occur when suffering from depression, injury, or debilitating anxiety.

The American Psychiatric Association points out the following valuable lessons connecting mental health issues to athletes. First, mental illness is very likely as common in athletes as in the general population. It is not a sign of weakness and should be taken as seriously as a physical injury. Getting help will most likely improve, not damage, one's self-confidence.

Lastly, remember that sports subject individuals to a unique set of challenges and circumstances that can make anyone vulnerable to feelings of depression or anxiety.

Interpersonal Issues with Teammates

Sport psychologists can also help resolve interpersonal issues within a team, or between an athlete and a coach. Whenever you need an open nonjudgmental, confidential platform to figure out a problem and understand it better, that's when you would seek a psychologist. For example, if your coach is bullying you or another member of your team, and you don't know how to appropriately respond to or handle the situation, a qualified sport psychologist can come in to help you resolve the problem. He or she can help clarify the situation so that the right decisions or policy can be made.

In a team setting, your club or organization would have to approve bringing in a sport psychologist. Or, you can work with one on your own to develop the correct language and mindset, which is particularly helpful when dealing with difficult individuals.

Treating Anxiety and Depression

Depression and anxiety are two different disorders that each require professional treatment. True depression or anxiety occurs when you are suffering from either for more than two weeks at a time, which is different than the occasional anxiety or blue mood, or a response to a specific life stressor. In these instances, you will be able to snap out of your funk or remove yourself from the situation. But if you find that you can't move on, or experience self-defeating thoughts, you may be suffering from depression or anxiety.

Mental health issues like depression can actually mask a physical health issue, which is one reason why it's so important to get a physical with all the blood work to make sure you're healthy. Unexplained depression might actually be a symptom of anemia, Lyme disease, or a traumatic brain injury. Symptoms of depression are also often confused with overtraining.

The following are some of the most common signs of depression:

- **Sleep changes:** increased during day or decreased sleep at night
- **Interest:** loss of interest in activities that used to interest them
- **Guilt:** feeling worthless
- **Energy (lack):** one of the most common presenting symptom is fatigue
- **Cognition/concentration:** reduced cognition and/or difficulty concentrating
- **Appetite:** changes in, resulting in weight gain or loss
- **Psychomotor:** agitation (anxiety) or retardations (lethargic)
- Suicide/death preoccupation

Anxiety can have some symptoms similar to those of depression, but there are distinct differences in its symptomatology. Those with true anxiety disorders frequently have intense, excessive and persistent worry and fear about everyday situations. Often, anxiety disorders involve repeated episodes of sudden feelings of intense anxiety, such as panic attacks. These feelings can interfere with daily activities, are difficult to control, are out of proportion to the actual danger, and can last a long time.

In athletes, anxiety can be caused by past negative experiences. While they might have receded into the background of our inner world, they continue to affect present thinking patterns. For example, past parental ridicule of childhood athletic performance can exert a detrimental influence if the athlete continues a pattern of negative self-talk based on those parental criticisms.

Eating Disorders

One of the things that is so appealing about elite athletes, and athletics in general, is how we look when we are active. However, when you see elite athletes and their perfectly chiseled bodies, remember that to some extent, they may come with a cost. Sadly, eating disorders are very common with athletes, affecting both men and women. In a study of Division I NCAA athletes, over a third of female athletes reported attitudes and symptoms that placed them at risk of anorexia. Athletes often struggle with eating disorders if their sport places emphasis on physical shape. However, it's important to remember that eating disorders do not occur because of sports; they are mind issues that include extreme emotions, attitudes, and behaviors surrounding weight and food issues.

A second issue athletes often face is referred to as *body dysmorphia*: a body-image disorder characterized by persistent and intrusive preoccupations with an imagined or slight defect in one's appearance. This issue is very common in sports where you have to show your physique, such as gymnastics, dance, body-building, or swimming. For these athletes, no matter what they see in the mirror, they focus on some imperfection. The result is that often, they start behaviors that are actually harmful, such as substance abuse.

As we look up to elite athletes who have perfect bodies as role models, keep in mind that their seemingly perfect bodies might be a sign that they're really not all that healthy. The fact is, elite athletes often have a high tendency for perfectionism. However, striving for perfection is different than perfectionism, especially when it is interfering with your quality of life. It's fine to be a perfectionist, as long as you're doing it in a safe and ethical way. You don't have to compromise your health to achieve your goals. Some of these elite athletes might have been trained poorly, or had a coach that gave them poor advice. The goal of this book is to make sure you don't fall into those traps.

Eating disorders needs to be addressed through professional mental health interventions. The most common among athletes include:

- **Anorexia:** Inadequate food intake accompanied by an intense fear of weight gain, obsession with weight, and persistent behavior to prevent weight gain.
- **Binge Eating Disorder:** Frequent episodes of consuming large amounts of food but without behaviors to prevent weight gain, such as self-induced vomiting. These episodes are accompanied by a feeling of being out of control.
- **Bulimia:** Frequent episodes of consuming large amounts of food followed by behaviors to prevent weight gain, such as self-induced vomiting. These episodes are accompanied by a feeling of being out of control.
- **Orthorexia:** An unhealthy obsession with otherwise healthy eating. Orthorexia starts out as an innocent attempt to eat more healthfully, but orthorexics become fixated on food quality and purity. Food choices become so restrictive, in both variety and calories, that health suffers.

CHAPTER 10
THE SPIRITUAL LEADER

I give all the glory to God. It's kind of a win-win situation. The glory goes up to him, and the blessings fall down on me.

—Gabby Douglas, US gymnast and 2012 Olympic Gold Medalist

In 2009 I was working as a physician for the California State Athletic Commission when I met a young, energetic boxer in San Diego. Covered in tattoos, he had crosses and religious quotes all over his body. He told me once that his faith in a higher power was what kept him focused on being the best boxer he could be. Draping a rosary around his neck after each win, he would proudly thank God for all he had accomplished.

His religious conviction got me curious as to how many athletes use spirituality as a motivator that might lead to better performance. Then I remembered my own high school experience, when Friday night football games were preceded by a Mass with Father Gulley. His sermon typically covered the topics of fair play, integrity, and how we were going to be victorious. At the end of every sermon he would bless us with his wish for safety and his hope that we should perform well. I wouldn't say Father Gulley's words led us to complete a 16–0 season every year, but they worked to connect the team on a deeper level, even though some of us, including myself, weren't even Catholic. I remember feeling that Father Gulley's words created a spiritual protection for us on the field; we knew that someone was protecting us from harm. His words also provided clarity regarding our true purpose: to play the best we could as a team.

This sense of purpose bonded us. We would leave the Mass with a sense of calm and resolve.

Today, when I'm on the tennis court and I feel connected to nature and to my spiritual self, I notice that my game improves. Whenever I'm double-faulting, or missing a few shots in a row, I stop for a second and I take my eyes off the court. I look around and take in my natural surroundings, and start to feel part of the spiritual world. Then I reflect back to the meaning of my endeavor, which is to play the best tennis I can whether I win or lose, and then I can get back in the game feeling a bit renewed.

The vast majority of the elite athletes that I've ever treated, interviewed, or just hung out with, have some belief in a higher power which they credit for increasing their performance. Organizations such as the Fellowship of Christian Athletes (FCA) and the Center for Sport and Jewish Life in America demonstrate the significant connection between religion and athletics. One of the unique features of the Olympics is the tradition of the host country creating a multi-faith center, placed right in the Athletes' Village.

At the player level, we've all seen professional athletes connect to their spiritual side directly on the court, track, football field, or baseball diamond. For example, the famous New York Yankee's closer Mariano Rivera is quoted as saying, "Everything I have and everything I became is because of the strength of the Lord, and through him I have accomplished everything. Not because of my strength. Only by His love, His mercy, and His strength."

Some players even embrace other practices than their own, especially when they are away from home. According to ESPN, during Wimbledon tournaments, Novak Djokovic finds an escape at the Buddhapadipa Temple to meditate and relieve stress between matches, even though Djokovic isn't Buddhist. However, he appreciates the serenity at the temple and enjoys getting away from the crowds and the opportunity to enjoy nature.

Over the years other elite athletes have shared with me that once they recognize they are only a small part of a bigger system, whether the system is their team, their overall sport, their community, or ultimately the world, they realize how their own efforts benefit more than just themselves. This sense of a greater purpose motivates them to perform better and contribute more to the team. They recognize that each member plays a distinct role, and like the various instruments in an orchestra, work together to create something entirely different than just their singular piece. What's more, by seeing how they fit into the bigger picture, it motivates them to perform at a level that could have never been accomplished individually.

Many of these elite athletes grew up in homes steeped in spirituality. As adults who can choose whether or not to include spirituality in their lives, I'm always amazed at how strongly they believe in a higher power. However, I shouldn't be so surprised; according to a Gallup poll, 95 percent of Americans believe in God. In fact, the vast majority of people in this world believe in a higher power.

In 2003, researcher Coakley found that spiritually focused athletes use prayer in six distinct ways. They may use prayer as a coping mechanism during stressful situations; to help guide a morally sound life; to dedicate their commitment to their particular sport; to put their athletic endeavors into perspective; to establish a strong bond of attachment between teammates; and to maintain social control. To me, spirituality is the ultimate connection that can provide peace, comfort, and a sense of purpose. When you fully understand your life's purpose, it's like uncovering your athletic mission statement. When you wrote your statement in Chapter One, you acknowledged the trajectory of your athletic path. As I've said earlier, just knowing that you have a mission and a goal allows you the freedom to pursue improving your game. The hesitation of the "why" you are following this particular path is removed, as well as the obstacles you may have put in your own way.

Bestselling author and leadership expert Ken Blanchard loves saying, "God don't make no junk," which means that we're each here on this earth for a reason. We're here for a purpose. There are many elite athletes who believe that their purpose is to use their talent and reach their maximum potential. Anything short of that would not be honoring their god. If they serve this role perfectly, it is consistent with their mission statement.

I've found that the athletes who live their purpose are actually the most grounded. They aren't anxious about their performance or overly competitive because they believe that whatever the outcome, just following their purpose adds to the greater good of the world. What's more, their sense of connectedness increases their ability to focus, and that resonates with teammates and opponents, as well as the rest of their entourage. If you can tap into this sense of connectedness others might take your skills and your focus more seriously, making you a more formidable opponent. You may also find that being connected to a bigger system allows you to be more aware of other people, too, which can help improve your game strategy.

Tapping into my spirituality helps me mentally recover from losing because I can take my emotions out of the moment and remember that even a loss is part of the bigger picture of winning. To err is human, and overcoming adversity is an expected and welcomed aspect of sports. We put ourselves out there as a test of our talents. Staying spiritually connected reminds us that no one is supposed to perform perfectly each time they enter a competition. How we handle errors is then the key to stepping up our game.

Once you recognize that you're part of a bigger system, you can look at each game, each competition, in the same light. You have one role to play, and if you trust that when you play your role, the other players will do what they're supposed to do, your team can perform at a higher level, greater than any one of the individual player's talents. This is in some sense the spirituality of team play.

Lastly, it is more the rule than the exception that elite athletes play with integrity and take responsibility for their actions. I've found that the athletes who embrace their spirituality are more apt to follow the rules and make better choices on and off the field. They may be guided by a good moral compass that comes from having a spiritual leader they trust. I believe that each of the world's religions instruct us to be the most noble person. Knowing that you are part of a community may help you stay on the right path, and avoid the temptations athletes face, such as performance enhancers or any type of cheating.

Time-Out: Athletes as Spiritual Leaders

According to the *New York Times*, some spiritually focused athletes take it a step further. Former Atlanta Hawks star Andrew Lang now volunteers as his former team's chaplain, taking prayer requests and speaking with players—of both the Hawks and the opposing team—who look for his guidance before each home game. Lang, who became a minister while he was still playing, attended pregame chapel services throughout his career, finding that they helped build his confidence and find his voice on the court.

The NBA's first chapel meeting dates back to 1979. Today, all thirty NBA teams have volunteer chaplains. One hour before every game, inside every arena, players from both sides are invited to attend a session that usually lasts fifteen minutes or less. For some players, attending chapel service has become a part of their pregame routine.

Meet NFL Superstar Ed White

Ed White began his professional football career with the Minnesota Vikings in 1969. He is one of just eleven players to have played in all four Vikings Super Bowl appearances. Later, he was traded to the San Diego Chargers, where he played until 1985, appearing in over 240 total games. Since retiring from the NFL, White has coached football for the

Chargers, the Rams, Cal State, and San Diego State. He has since been inducted into College Football Hall of Fame, the University of California Hall of Fame, and the San Diego Charger Hall of Fame.

When I interviewed Ed, he told me that spirituality was a constant presence in his life, and how he was able to use it to be a very aggressive player. "I was raised in a southern Baptist church. My father was a non-practicing Hungarian Jew from Virginia. He married my mother, an Irish Catholic lady who became a southern Baptist. My mother was a very spiritual woman. She loved everyone. It was wonderful thing to grow up in that environment. They passed their religion onto me, and I've passed it on to my children and grandchildren.

"I really try to balance my spirituality and the physical part of my life. When I was a professional football player, I mixed spirituality with visualization techniques. I just feel blessed; visualization was something that I have in me, which inhabits me. It became a real part of my life in terms of how I was successful on the field. Now I use visualization to become a better artist. My art is focused on my spirituality.

"As a player I sometimes visualized myself as an airplane bomber, or as a gladiator in ancient times. I felt like I was down there on the colosseum floor fighting for my life. But the spirit that I most often competed with was more of a wild horse. The complexity of that spirit is that wild horses are fighters who want to dominate and take the will to compete away from their opponent. In my psyche I was going to be a wild man from the first play until the last one. I was playing as hard as I could on every down. At some point, my opponent would start thinking, 'This guy is crazy. He's going to play like this the whole game. I might as well give up now.' And amazingly, many times, my opponent was slowed down by my wild horse spirit.

"I believe that athletes who are spiritually connected see life as energy, and see it as a continuing energy that moves on, even when the physical existence is over. When my daughter passed away when she was only eighteen—just one week past her high school graduation—I would go

251

into her room. There was still a mobile over her bed, and I would sit in her room and talk to her for days afterward, and every time I started talking, that mobile would start spinning around. That's the energy that flows in us, that doesn't die. There is no doubt in my mind. I've seen it, I know it.

"I think that what spiritually based athletes have is that enlightenment, that wisdom of knowing that that energy exists, and you can tap into it to become a more powerful person, mentally, spiritually, and physically."

Developing Your Spiritual Side

Within their entourage, elite athletes all have their own version of a spiritual leader. It can be a person of faith, or it might be someone who makes them feel the connection to a larger community, however they define it. A spiritual leader should not be judgmental toward others, or think that "their way" is better than others. They don't denounce other faiths, and come to their religious teachings from a place of love, not from punishment, and certainly not fear. If you already have a religious institution that you belong to, and you haven't been there in a while, maybe that's something to look at. Set up a meeting with your spiritual leader, and see how the pursuit of sports fits in with their teachings.

Don't be embarrassed if you haven't attended services for a while. As we grow up, we often cast our spiritual self aside, rebelling against our parents' or our community's beliefs. I know I certainly rebelled when I was young. I started exploring other religions, and eventually realized their singular beauty: for me, all religions are the same. They just provide different tools to get to the same message.

Even if you aren't a religious person, you can connect with your spiritual self. On my spiritual journey I also learned that religion is not necessarily spirituality. It certainly can be a means, but you can also feel connected sitting in nature, enjoying the sun, or experiencing something bigger than we could accomplish, such as art. I often find spiritual inspiration through others, even if they are not spiritual themselves. It can be anyone who brings out the best in you. For example, during the 2013 Super Bowl, I watched the winning coach of the Baltimore Ravens hand over the game ball to a former player who was now wheelchair-bound: O.J. Brigance. O.J. was one of the toughest players on the team a decade earlier. Unfortunately, he was diagnosed with ALS (a brain degenerative disease), but was such a smart player he took a front office strategic position. Still, he was the most prominent behind the scenes force for the Super Bowl–winning team, and was also considered to be the spiritual leader of the Ravens. The way he conducted himself while facing his limitations inspired the team to unite and feel connected.

Spirituality Exercise: Find Your Muse

There's a reason why religious services are steeped in music: it's an easy connection to the divine that anyone can harness. You might not think of your pregame soundtrack as a religious experience, but it is. Music can bring out the best in you by getting you motivated and mentally focused. For game days, start listening to your soundtrack about an hour prior to the game. You can also create a different playlist for your pregame warm-up and daily workouts.

You can also tap into your spiritual self through the music of prayer. Prior to going on the field, find a prayer that resonates with you. It doesn't have to be religious but if you have a favorite one that you remember, use it. If not, ask your religious leader for some suggestions, or look for poems that inspire you. You can also ask some of your older teammates, or players you know for suggestions that have worked for them.

Here's an example of a prayer I often recommend to my patients:

May I compete with love shining in my heart. May I push myself to be the best athlete I believe I can be. May I have the strength, courage, endurance and skills I will need. May I put into practice all that I have learned in training, and bring to mind all my preparation. May I remember the goodness in my life, and may this goodness pour out of me.

Sit with this prayer, one of your own, or even a poem for just a few minutes before your game. If you can memorize it, you can use it as a strategy to motivate yourself to play to your best abilities.

I've heard that in professional football, the last thing the players do before they take the field is say a prayer together. The head coach typically brings his team into a loose huddle in the locker room and everyone takes a knee, holds hands and bows their heads. Then, the entire team recites the Lord's Prayer. Whether you are religious or not, this is a very effective way to unite the players.

Pregame Meditation

Meditation provides you with the tools to connect with something larger than yourself. What's more, meditation has been shown to help in areas that could relate to athletic performance. First, meditation has been shown to increase your ability to focus, and when you are in pain, it can help you cope by redirecting your attention. Meditation has been shown to calm the fear center of the brain even when you're not meditating, and helps reset the mind to focus on the present, especially if you fall victim to negative self-talk. It reduces stress, pregame jitters, nervousness, and anxiety, and teaches you how to quiet your emotions. When athletes relax, energy flows more freely throughout the body, greatly improving your capability to perform.

Practice meditating every day. Find a comfortable place where you can be alone. Turn off all technology. Sit down and close your eyes, and for the first few minutes focus on your breath. Then, let your mind go, without judgment, and once you feel your mind wander slowly bring your focus back to your breath. Continue to do this loop for ten minutes, and add a few more minutes as necessary, building up to thirty minutes a day if possible.

Once you get comfortable with mediation, you can add a visualization, just as Ed White did. The simplest way to learn to visualize is to look straight ahead and then close your eyes. See how much you can recall of what you had just been looking at. Repeatedly opening and shutting the eyes and trying to visualize more of the scene will prove to you that practice does increase your ability to recall the image.

When you have mastered this basic visualization, start to picture in your mind's eye a mental picture of what it looks like when you are achieving your goals. What spirit or energy do you connect with? Is it an animal, a force, or another type of object? Fill in as many details as possible. If you have difficulty creating your own mental picture, find one in a magazine or on the Internet that inspires you. Hold that image in your hand, or in your mind, for a two full minutes.

Getting In The Zone

I have found that when we enjoy what we are doing with purpose, time passes effortlessly. The Tao Te Ching describes this feeling as being one with "The Way." When there is a synchronization of one's effort with their true purpose, the effort does not feel much like work but rather more like "being in the moment."

For example, when I ran the Rock 'n' Roll Marathon in 2006, at mile twenty-three I suddenly felt strangely connected with my surroundings. After that, every step forward felt like an "effortless effort," or "being in the zone." I believe this feeling comes from connecting with your deeper spiritual self. It is a joy that can be tapped when one has their Way, or purpose, realized.

In Ed White's interview, his effortless effort took place when he could connect with his visualization of the wild horse. It was almost like he would feel this force come through him, which is what gave him the advantage on the football field. Many athletes will talk like that about their performance. They'll say, "Today's game was just effortless. I felt connected and had a clear energy and passion and accuracy. I don't know where that came from, but I'm grateful for it."

CHAPTER 11
CREATING A UNIFIED PROGRAM

I am a member of a team, and I rely on the team, I defer to it and sacrifice for it, because the team, not the individual, is the ultimate champion.

—Mia Hamm

By now you should have a complete understanding of everything you need to do to step up your game, no matter what sport or activity you are pursuing. You've learned exactly how to live and train like an elite athlete. You've explored each role in the entourage and can see why each is unique yet necessary, and that in order to achieve peak performance you need to make sure that you are following their best practices. The last step is integrating them into one seamless program.

Adopting each of these roles can be easily worked into your current routine. The truth is, not every one of the roles needs to be attended to every day. The following chart will show exactly how often you need to think about each role. Of course, there will be plenty of days that you are attending to several at one time. I hope that you find, as I have, that the more you think about each of these roles, the easier it is to adopt their strategies, and the more you get out of the entire program.

Now that you fully understand these roles you have in effect made them available to you, so that they will be accessible whenever you need them. The last thing you want is to start researching a specific role in a time of crisis. Instead, you can relax a bit, knowing that every aspect of your training has been taken care of. And when emergencies or glitches occur, and we know that they will, you will be all the more prepared to deal with them.

The Step Up Your Game Checklist

The Athletic Mission Statement and Goals: Review your athletic mission statement every six months, and check in with your individual goals each month. You can also check in with either whenever you feel you are losing faith in your game or going through a losing streak or decreased performance. At your season's end, reassess your goals and see if you want to continue on to next season. And of course, whenever you meet your goals, don't waste too much time setting new ones.

Team Physician: You will need an annual physical. If you starting a new routine, check in with your doctor at least four-to-six weeks prior to beginning training (allow more lead time if you have chronic medical conditions). This will provide enough time to resolve any condition or ailment found during the physical. For example, if your doctor finds a heart murmur on the physical exam, there is enough time to get an ultrasound to see if it is anything to be concerned about. You can also consider checking in quarterly or as needed if injury or illness occurs.

Physical therapist: During preseason and in season training you will be doing your prehabilitation at least two-to-three times per week. When you are out of season you can cut back to following a weekly routine.

Trainer: Daily, both in and out of season. On this program you will be doing some form of training daily, with the obligatory day off.

Dietitian: Daily both in and out of season. On this program you will be following this eating plan every single day. Remember, diet is the single most important preventive approach to healthy living, regardless of your athletic pursuits.

Coach: Daily, in-season; once a month off-season. It is important to keep checking in with your self-coach in the off-season so you can keep track of your goals.

Competitor: During game days in-season, and when you feel the need for extra motivation during practice. Let go of your competitor in the off-season to make room for new ones next year.

Role Model: Weekly during season, monthly off-season. In the off-season thinking about your role model, or finding new ones, can keep you out of trouble when things are not so structured.

Psychologist: Training the brain is as important as training the body. Daily in-season; weekly off-season. As needed during times of stress, anxiety, depression.

Spiritual Leader: Weekly and before each game. Once a month in the off-season. Also as needed during times of stress, anxiety, and depression.

The Step Up Your Game Checklist					
	Yearly	Half-Yearly	Monthly	Weekly	Daily
Athletic Mission Statement		X			
Goals			X		
Team Physician	X		X-4–6 weeks prior to starting a new routine		
Physical Therapist				X-off season	X-in season
Trainer					X

	Yearly	Half-Yearly	Monthly	Weekly	Daily
Dietitian					X
Coach			X- off-season		X-in-season
Competitor				X-every game	
Role Model			X- off-season	X- in-season	
Psychologist				X-off-season	X-in-season
Spiritual Leader			X- off-season	X- in-season	

Chart Your Progress

On a regular calendar mark when you are supposed to check in with each of the roles according to the checklist, and then keep good records. You can even set reminders on your phone. For example, if your annual physical is supposed to be in six months (which is six weeks prior to the beginning of your season), put a reminder to call your doctor in three months so that you have a physical six weeks prior to the beginning of your season.

I have found, time and again, that if you don't keep up with the checklist, it is the most likely cause of decreased performance or not achieving your goals. If you have not been diligent with keeping up with your checklist, discuss it with your sports physician. There will always be a tweak to your plan and your physician will be able to direct you to which role needs to be adjusted, or may recommend getting professional help if that particular role may be deficient.

Success On and Off the Field

Living like an elite athlete can set you up for any type of success. When retired Olympic athletes have to join the rest of us in the working world, they're highly attractive prospects. Employers respect that these athletes know what stiff competition is like. They know how to handle pressure, and they know to settle for nothing less than their absolute best effort. What's more, they know how to be advised and take constructive criticism. They know what to do when failure occurs. In short, they can conquer any obstacle in front of them.

The principles in this book can be applied to anyone looking to lead a balanced, high performance life. I have been using this concept for many years in my practice, and found that it works well as a framework for all types of people beyond my athletes, including executives, employers, parents, entrepreneurs, performers, etc. Whenever a patient comes to me and asks, "How do I have a better relationship with my wife?" or "I want to lose weight" or "I want to get a promotion at my company" or "I want to excel at my trade," I refer them to this methodology. We look at these questions as a set of new challenges, just like an athlete would. Then, we review each of the roles and see how they would help tackle that challenge, and how to incorporate them into their life.

I hope you'll share this program with your family so that everyone can benefit. And keep these teachings in mind even after you've played your last game. You can then impart your secrets to great performance onto others, paying it forward. Be the example for others—there is nothing more rewarding than being a part of someone else's success in stepping up their game.

REFERENCES

Alter, D.A., M. O'Sullivan, P.I. Oh, et al. "Synchronized Personalized Music Audio-playlists to Improve Adherence to Physical Activity among Patients Participating in a Structured Exercise Program: A Proof-ofprinciple Feasibility Study." *Sports Medicine—Open* 1(1) (2015):23. doi:10.1186/s40798–015-0017–9.

Baker, J., J. Cote, and R. Hawes. "The Relationship between Coaching Behaviours and Sport Anxiety in Athletes." *Journal of Science and Medicine in Sport* 3(2) (June 2000):110–119.

Berkman, Seth. "Cornell's Chocolate Milk Fills Refueling Gap." *New York Times,* April 18, 2015. http://www.nytimes.com/2015/04/19/sports/cornells-chocolate-milk-fills-refueling-gap.html   Braverman, Eric R. *Younger (thinner) You Diet: How Understanding Your Brain Chemistry Can Help You Lose Weight, Reverse Aging, and Fight Disease.* New York: Rodale, 2009.

Coakley, Jay. *Sports in Society,* 8th ed. Boston: Irwin McGraw-Hill, 2003.

Cobb, Laura K., Job G. Godino, Elizabeth Selvin, Anna Kucharska-Newton, Josef Coresh, and Silvia Koton. "Physical Activity among Married Couples in the Atherosclerosis Risk in Communities (ARIC) Study." *Circulation* 131 (2015): AP275.

Feltz, D.L., M.A. Chase, S.E. Moritz, and P.J. Sullivan. "A Conceptual Model of Coaching Efficacy: Preliminary Investigation and Instrument Development." *Journal of Educational Psychology* 91 (1999): 675–776.

Karageorghis, Costas I. "Music-Based Interventions." *In Encyclopedia of Sport and Exercise Psychology,* edited by Robert C. Eklund and Gershon Tenenbaum. Thousand Oaks, CA: Sage, 2014.

Kato, Kim, Stephanie Jevas, and Dean Culpepper. "Body Image Disturbances in NCAA Division I and III Female Athletes." *The Sports Journal*, United States Sports Academy, September 30, 2011. http://thesportjournal.org/article/body-image-disturbancesin-ncaa-division-i-and-iii-female-athletes

Life, Jeffry S. *The Life Plan: How Any Man Can Achieve Lasting Health, Great Sex, and a Stronger, Leaner Body.* New York: Atria, 2011.

Marx, J.O., et al. "Low-Volume Circuit versus High-Volume Periodized Resistance Training in Women." *Medicine & Science in Sports & Exercise* 33 (2001): 635–643.

Mitchell, J.H., W. Haskell, P. Snell, and S.P. Van Camp. "Task Force 8: Classification of Sports." *Journal of the American College of Cardiology* 45 (2005): 1364–1367.

Rice et al. *Pediatrics.* Medical Conditions Affecting Sports Participation. 121: 4 April 2008.

Riley, Pat. *The Winner Within: A Life Plan for Team Players.* New York: Putnam's Sons, 1993.

Reynolds, Gretchen. "Should Athletes Eat Fat or Carbs?" *New York Times,* February 25, 2015. http://well.blogs.nytimes.com/2015/02/25/shouldathletes-eat-fat-or-carbs/?_r=0

Volek, J.S., T. Noakes, S.D. Phinney. "Rethinking Fat as a Fuel for Endurance Exercise." *European Journal of Sport Science* 15(1) (2015):13–20. doi: 10.1080/17461391.2014.959564. Epub 2014 Oct 2.

APPENDIX

Consumer Resources

The following websites and related ideas are excellent resources for finding professionals for many of the roles in your elite athlete entourage:

The Team Physician:
American Osteopathic Academy of Sports Medicine: www.aoasm.org - go to 'find a sports medicine DO'

American Medical Society for Sports Medicine: www.amssm.org - go to 'find a sports doc'

American College of Osteopathic Family Physicians: www.acofp.org - go to 'find a physician'

American Board of Family Medicine: www.theabfm.org - go to 'find a physician'

The Physical Therapist:
American Physical Therapy Association: www.apta.org - go to 'find a PT'

Ask your physician to recommend a local PT

Your team may have an athletic trainer; talk to your coach

The Trainer:
American College of Sports Medicine: ACSM members.acsm.org/source/custom/Online_locator/OnlineLocator.cfm

select at certification/registry level- 'ACSM certified personal trainer'

American Council on Exercise: ACE www.acefitness.org/acefit/locate-trainer/

IDEA Health and Fitness Association www.ideafit.com/ select find a trainer

National Strength and Conditioning Association: NSCA www.nsca.com/Membership/Member-Tools/Find-a-Trainer/

The Dietitian:

Academy of Nutrition and Dietetics: www.eatright.org/find-an-expert -select 'find an expert'

The Coach:

Find local club for sport: www.coachup.com

The Psychologist:

Association for Applied Sport Psychology: www.appliedsportpsych.org/ - select 'find a consultant'

ACKNOWLEDGMENTS

This herculean feat has been the result of being fortunate to meet the right people at the right time. First and foremost I want to thank my wife Sneha, the heart of our family, who has allowed me to be who I am meant to be. As many have said when I first introduced her to my family over fifteen years ago, "Naresh, don't screw this up!" My fantastically dynamic and lovely daughter, Jasmine, known as J. J. G. (Jazzy Jaz Girl) to her friends, teaches me to be forever playful. My quick-witted and energetic son, Arjun, shows me how to see the world through renewed eyes, especially during our hikes. I am blessed with two sets of parents, Jyothi and Govind Rao and Sarswati and Vajubhai Sanchala, who have been unconditionally supportive as I fulfill my dreams. My "consigliere" and brother-in-law, Tejash Sanchala, is always there to guide me through the legal side of any venture I undertake. My cousin, Lokesh Rao, has always been like a kid brother and hitting partner in tennis, letting me get the stress out on the court when I need it most. I am also thankful to my brother, Sonny Rao, for allowing us to grow closer over the past few years. Many thanks for the technical computer support from the original "little guy," Neil Sanchala. And to my dearest Samina Rao and Kieran Malloy-Good Sanchala, the newest additions to our growing family, thanks for keeping me feeling forever young.

The idea of this book became a reality through the most amazingly gifted writer who I had the pure dumb luck of meeting one fine Sunday afternoon. Pam Liflander's wisdom, experience, and witty demeanor kept the momentum going full force, and I am eternally grateful to have her in my life. My agent, Carol Mann, to whom Pam introduced me, gave me the opportunity of a lifetime by agreeing to represent me and find a publisher for this book. Many thanks to Niels Aaboe and the folks at Sports Publishing for believing in this book.

Thank you Betsey Armstrong, Tucker Dupree, Joe Hippensteel, Wendy Hilliard, Roch Frey, Heather Fuhr, Shawn Heuglin, Adam Krikorian, Dean Reinmuth, Peter Holmberg, Tony Azevedo, Dr. Burt Giges, and Ed White for taking your precious time for the interviews. You have all enriched my life and will undoubtedly enrich the lives of everyone who reads this book.

A special thanks to Sabrina Zaslov, MS, RD/N, CDE for her assistance with creating the nutrition meal plan, and Anthony Darmiento for reviewing the physical therapist and trainer chapters and providing his strength and conditioning expertise. Also, I loved the experience of having two of the best fitness models, Freddie Kimmel and Becca Pace, being photographed by the efficient and professional Matt Simpkins.

I have been inspired by many physicians who taught me the art of medicine. My father was the first to go to college in our family, and became a doctor, moving to the United States from India with just two suitcases in the 1960s. He taught me that applying passion and determination to anything can lead to extraordinary results. Dr. Michael Sheridan introduced me to family medicine and showed me how special it is to care for our patients with compassion. Dr. Martha Lansing was my program director during residency and brought out the "Family Doc" in me. Dr. Richard Levandowski, my first sports medicine mentor, opened my eyes to what my true calling is and gave me a taste of the amazing field of primary care sports medicine. Dr. Lee Rice took me under his wing and showed me the highest level of service a doctor can offer through sports medicine and corporate wellness—thank you for making me not only a better doctor but a better person. Dr. Rick Parker showed me how to be a leader in primary care sports medicine and the meaning being a true friend. Dr. Marcia Whalen gave me my big break by introducing me to USA Water Polo.

Dr. Cliff Stark, my senior resident and today one of my partners at Sports Medicine at Chelsea, showed me the passion for this field and has been a true friend. My other partner, Dr. Aran Degenhardt, helped me understand that family medicine can be combined holistically with other medical systems, such as traditional Chinese medicine, and be innovative. Thanks to our staff of physical therapists, physician assistants, and office administrators for their support and for taking excellent care of our patients. And speaking of my patients, thank you from the bottom of my heart for the gift of allowing me to be enriched by your trust—it is an honor and privilege to care for each and every one of you.

Mary Rice showed me what true empathy and caring are all about, and I always keep that close to my heart. Thanks to the American Osteopathic Academy of Sports Medicine for the camaraderie in sharing a vision that is in alignment with my true purpose.

Thanks to USA Water Polo for allowing me to serve the players, and for making my own Olympic dreams come true. Thanks to the New York Athletic Club for inviting me to be part of the water polo club, to help mold the Olympians of tomorrow through coaching, and simply for being my home away from home.

To my "West Hall" crew, Class of 1993 Colgate University, thank you for your true friendship—I love that we keep rockin' it every year together. Thanks to my NYITCOM medical school buddies Dr. Prem Chattoo, Dr. Vijai Tivakaran, and Dr. Medhi Khan—you are my friends for life. To the Chattoo family, thank you for being my family away from home. Thanks to Eleanor Jaffe for being so supportive during my transition back to NY. And thanks to Quan Campbell, co-founder of the Lifewellness Institute, for coaching me across the finish line at the San Diego Rock'n'Roll Marathon.

I'll always remember Dr. J. Zink and his wise advice prior to leaving San Diego, "Write your book brother." Many thanks to Marika and Neil Bender for their support—you both gave this book a chance to make it. Thanks to the amazingly gifted screen writer, Kranti Pally, for his advice and support through this process. Last but not least, I owe a debt of gratitude to Michael Morrison—without his enthusiasm this book would never have been written.

INDEX